Parkinson's Disease

300 Tips for Making Life Easier

By
Shelley Peterman Schwarz

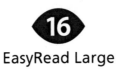

16

EasyRead Large

RHYW

Copyright Page from the Original Book

Demos Medical Publishing, LLC
386 Park Avenue South, Suite 301
New York, NY 10016

Visit our website at www.demosmedpub.com

Library of Congress Cataloging-in-Publication Data

Schwarz, Shelley Peterman.
   Parkinson's disease : 300 tips for making life easier / Shelley Peterman Schwarz.—2nd ed.
      p.   cm.
   Includes index.
   ISBN-10: 1-932603-53-0
   ISBN-13: 978-1932-60353-8
   1. Parkinson's disease—Popular works.   I. Title.

   RC382.S3825   2006
   616.8'33—dc22

                                                                            2005031761

Manufactured in the United States of America

06   07   08   09   10   5   4   3   2   1

RHYW

TABLE OF CONTENTS

Dedication   i

A Word from the Author   iii

CHAPTER 1: Basic Concepts for Living with Parkinson's Disease   1

CHAPTER 2: Making Your Home Safe and Accessible   19

CHAPTER 3: Looking Good, Feeling Better   54

CHAPTER 4: Communicating   73

CHAPTER 5: Managing Mealtime Madness   95

CHAPTER 6: Empowering Yourself   121

CHAPTER 7: Handling Medical Issues   154

CHAPTER 8: Getting Out and About   188

About the Author   211

Index   213

Dedication

To Judy Ross, my mentor, cheerleader, and dear friend: Thank you for believing in me!

To Ina Sharkansky, my quiet, unwavering supporter: Thank you for your kindness and friendship.

To Deborah Proctor, my right arm and able assistant: Thank you for all your hard work!

To my husband, David: There are no words to adequately thank you for giving me the freedom to live my life to the fullest. YOU are a remarkable man!

To all my wonderful friends and neighbors: please know that I couldn't do what I do without you, and you have my deepest, heartfelt thanks.

Resources marked with (*) are found in the Resources section at the end of each chapter.

Throughout this book you will notice tips with the (**) designation. These tips are especially for people who provide care and support for people with PD.

A Word from the Author

Dear Reader:

It is my pleasure to present the second edition of *Parkinson's Disease: 300 Tips for Making Life Easier.* This updated and expanded edition is filled with tried-and-true tips, techniques, shortcuts, and resources that will help people coping with Parkinson's disease (PD). These simple, inexpensive hints will save you time and energy, lessen your frustration, and promote safety and independence.

The information for this book was gathered from two sources: (1) interviews with more than 100 people living with Parkinson's disease, people who care for people with PD, and healthcare professionals; and (2) my own personal experiences living with multiple sclerosis (MS), which, like Parkinson's disease, is a chronic, degenerative, and incurable illness.

Did you find it a shock when you or your friend or loved one was diagnosed with PD? When I was diagnosed with MS more than 25 years ago, it changed my life forever. My diagnosis came after years of minor but ever-present complaints. Frankly, when the diagnosis came, I was relieved that a name existed for my seemingly unrelated symptoms. And, for a few years, I tried to ignore the disease and pass as "normal." Eventually, my limitations became more serious, and I had to come to terms with the fact that I had a progressively degenerative disease that would have an impact not just on me but my family and friends as well.

Over the years, I've learned to incorporate into my life some basic concepts that have helped me immensely, and I've learned thousands of simple, time- and energy-saving tips that make a big difference in the quality of my life. Talking to others with chronic illnesses and disabilities has taught me a lot about survival and the human spirit and how strong and resilient people can be. We may not have a choice about having an illness, but we do have a choice in how we react to it.

Receiving a diagnosis such as Parkinson's disease can be distressing, and adjusting to the effects of the disease can be difficult, but you can still lead a remarkably unlimited life if you put your mind to it. By adapting your routine, making your home more accessible, and keeping a positive outlook, you have the power to take control of your life and rise above the challenges of PD.

This second edition of *Parkinson's Disease: 300 Tips for Making Life Easier* has been updated and expanded to include more tips to help you streamline daily activities, find ways to stay involved and in touch, and discover local, state, and national resources to make your life easier. For easy reference, the book is arranged in categories of daily activities. At the beginning of each chapter, I share some of the insights and observations people with PD have made while living with this disease. At the end of each chapter I have compiled a list of support organizations and providers of unique products that may make your life easier. Resources marked with (*) in the chapter are found in this resource section.

It is my hope that learning how other people deal with the challenges of Parkinson's disease will help you keep a positive attitude on your journey. I also hope the book will allow you to face the future with a sense of empowerment and control over the illness.

If, after reading this book, you would like to share your own Making Life Easier tips, or you would like to talk, I can be reached at www.M eetingLifesChallenges.com and at Shelley@Me etingLifesChallenges.com.

I wish you the best on your journey.

Shelley Peterman Schwarz

Other Books by Shelley

- *Blooming Where You're Planted: Stories from the Heart* (Meeting Life's Challenges, LLC, 1997, 2005)

- *Dressing Tips and Clothing Resources for Making Life Easier* (Attainment Company, 2000)

- *Multiple Sclerosis: 300 Tips for Making Life Easier* (Demos Medical Publishing, 1999, 2005)

- *Parkinson's Disease: 300 Tips for Making Life Easier* (Demos Medical Publishing, 2002, 2006)

- *Organizing Your IEPs* (Individualized Educational Plan for Special Education Students) (Attainment Company, 2005)

- *Memory: Tips for Making Life Easier* (Attainment Company, 2006)

Books with Shelley's Stories

- *Jewish Mothers Tell Their Stories: Acts of Love and Courage* (The Haworth Press, Inc., 2000)

- *Amazingly Simple Lessons We Learned After 50* (M. Evans and Co., Inc., 2001)

- *A Second Chicken Soup for the Woman's Soul* (Health Communications, Inc., 1998)

CHAPTER 1

Basic Concepts for Living with Parkinson's Disease

Being diagnosed with a chronic progressive illness like Parkinson's disease (PD) changes your life forever. Don't give up or give in to the disease! Today is a very hopeful time for people with PD. I hope these thoughts and observations will help you.

Staying Positive While Living with Parkinson's Disease

1. **Learn about your illness.** Don't be afraid to read about Parkinson's disease or talk to others who have it. Remember that no two cases are exactly alike, and no one can predict exactly how the disease will progress or affect *you.* Likewise, no two people respond exactly the same to treatments and medications. Gathering information about your illness, through books, medical journals, and the Internet, will empower you to make informed decisions about your medical care and the treatment options open to you. If you don't have In-

ternet access at home, visit your local library and ask a librarian how to visit helpful web sites.*

See if there is a Parkinson's disease or movement disorder clinic in your area. Many advances have been made in the treatment of PD. General neurologists may not be able to keep up to date on all areas of neurology; one who specializes in PD can confirm your diagnosis, review your medications, and consult with your primary care physician on your treatment.

Once you understand your illness, you are in a better position to take responsibility for your healthcare.

2.   **Look for ways to reduce your stress level and put yourself and your needs first.** This is not selfish or self-centered; you *must* take care of yourself first! You are the authority regarding your own body. Rest when you're tired. Be protective about how you spend your time and energy; Parkinson's disease uses a great deal of one's physical energy. Coping and adapting takes a great deal of emotional and mental energy. Do those things that are important to you and your family.

Give yourself permission to say "No," and not feel guilty. When you are feeling better, you can say "Yes."

3. **Try not to be self-conscious about the visible symptoms of your Parkinson's disease.** It may be challenging, but look for ways to work around the problems. If you are self-conscious about the way you walk, consider using a wheelchair. If hand tremors make it difficult to eat with utensils, and you feel embarrassed eating in a restaurant, order foods you can eat with your hands. Ask the waitress to put each item on a separate plate or bowl; that way your tremors are less likely to knock food off the plate. Don't let your visible symptoms of PD diminish the enjoyment you get from spending time with your family and friends. They love you for who you are and understand.

4. **Keep your sense of humor!** Having trouble walking, being unable to talk as loudly as you want, or giving up driving are not particularly funny. However, try to put a humorous spin on everyday observations and situations. For example, if you use a wheelchair, you might look at it this way: You always have a place to

sit and a pair of shoes lasts you 20 years. Remember, laughter is a great stress reducer.

5. **Surround yourself with caring, loving, and nurturing family members, friends, neighbors, and co-workers.** Give yourself permission to eliminate people and activities that drain your energy. Be honest with your family and friends if you're having a bad day. Explain that you may feel terrible in the morning but fine in the afternoon. Don't expect people to know what you are feeling unless you tell them.

6. **Tell people about your illness.** At any age, it can be difficult to share your feelings with your friends. And, it can be especially difficult if you're diagnosed with PD when you're young. Your friends may not know what PD is and may not know what to say or do—so tell them. Also, tell your hair stylist, dentist, and customer service people (as appropriate) that you may shake, lose your balance, move slowly, or have difficulties speaking because of PD. Ask for their help when you need it. People feel good when they can do something for someone else.

You might also want to keep a few informational brochures in your purse or wallet because you never know who might be interested in learning more about Parkinson's disease.

7. **Try to keep a positive attitude.** Even though it can be extremely difficult, as your symptoms change and the effectiveness of medications plays havoc with your life, look for the silver lining. It's perfectly natural to mourn the loss of function and independence for a brief time, but try not to get stuck there, wallow in self-pity, or isolate yourself from friends.

If you experience any combination of these symptoms—loss of appetite, feelings of sadness, difficulty sleeping, loss of your sense of humor, a sense of hopelessness, or just feel down in the dumps—you may be suffering from clinical depression. Please! Tell your doctor. Even though you have every right to be depressed about your diagnosis, depression is a treatable condition. A combination of antidepressants and/or psychotherapy can help lift your spirits and give you renewed energy to keep that allimportant positive attitude.

Remember: Your family and friends are not trained professionals. In fact, they may also be hurting because of your diagnosis. Perhaps they, too, could benefit from talking to someone about their fears and frustrations.

Listen to audiotapes and/or read books that promote positive thinking and deliver a healing message. The public library and bookstores offer an array of these materials.

8. **Set priorities and focus on tasks that must be done.** Tackle one job at a time. Break down activities into a series of smaller steps, and ask others to assist you with the difficult portions of the task. Avoid working or sitting for long periods in the same position. Move around periodically.

9. **Allow extra time to do everything** from eating, drinking, and dressing to walking, talking, and writing. Recognize that everything seems to take longer when you have Parkinson's disease. You'll also find that simple tasks most people take for granted, like swallowing saliva, chewing food, changing facial expressions, and projecting your voice, now require conscious thought. Plan to do activities around those times

when your medication gives you the most benefit. Mornings are often a better time of day to exercise and work because you are not as fatigued as in the afternoon. Although you may get fatigued during the day, be careful not to nap too much; otherwise, sleeping at night may be difficult. Taking a short nap after lunch can be revitalizing, but try to limit your daytime sleep so that your nighttime sleep can be more restful.

10. **Consider attending a local PD support group,** no matter what your age. Support group members understand your struggles because they face or have faced the same challenges. To find a Parkinson's disease support group in your community, see the Resources section at the end of this chapter or consult the Yellow Pages of your telephone book.

If you are reluctant to attend a PD support group because you will see others with advanced cases, and you don't think you can handle that, talk on the phone with others who have PD. Or, start a small group that gets together for lunch or coffee. Being with others who have PD may alleviate fears rather than worsen them. It is encouraging to see people with PD still driving, working, and caring for their families.

11. **Contact your local Independent Living Center (ILC).** Every community in the United States is part of a national network of independent living centers. More than 500 community-based, nonprofit ILCs serve people of all ages and disabilities and their families. Their goals are to provide information and referral, advocacy, peer support, and independent living skills training. These centers can: (1) Assist you in finding out about disability services in your community; (2) connect you with others to advocate for changes in the law or rules; (3) help you hire and manage personal care attendants; and (4) put you in contact with people who have faced challenges similar to your own.*

12. **Understand that it is common to have fluctuations in your mobility and energy levels during the day.** Often, these fluctuations coincide with when you take your medications, with the most fatigue and the least mobility coming as the medication wears off.

13. **Be willing to change the way you do things.** Remain flexible. Compromise. Accept the help that is offered and accept that more than one way exists to wash the dishes, put on clothes, or get from here to there. Practice patience—with yourself and others.

14. **Ask your doctor to prescribe evaluations by an occupational therapist (OT) and physical therapist (PT).** An OT will help you discover new ways of doing simple, everyday tasks like dressing, eating, and cooking. He can show you how to simplify your work and daily activities and conserve your energy. A PT will help you with mobility and home accessibility. Ask for a home evaluation, and ask the OT and PT to make suggestions for making your home and daily activities safer, more accessible, and easier to manage.

15. **Always try out any mobility equipment before you buy it.** That includes canes, walkers, manual and electric wheelchairs, transport chairs (all four of the wheels are the same size), and three-wheeled scooter

wheelchairs. Check out the size, weight, and ease of operation. If someone will be pushing your wheelchair, explain to that person about "courtesies of the road," including speed, cornering, handling leg rests, backing into elevators, going up and down curbs, and the like. (You will find more information about mobility aids in Chapter 6: Empowering Yourself.)

If you are considering purchasing a three- or four-wheeled scooter or wheelchair, find one that is easy to transport. Some chairs are lightweight and disassemble easily; others may require a lift that picks up the chair and puts it into the vehicle with minimal physical effort. Some automobile manufacturers, like Ford and Toyota, offer discounts and/or rebates for the purchase of adaptive equipment for people with disabilities. Ask your dealer about options and programs available.

16. **Make exercise part of your life.** Exercise does not reverse or delay the symptoms of PD, but it does help you make full use of your potential and improve your quality of life. It also helps prevent complications, such as contractures of rigid, poorly moving limbs. Walking, swimming, range-of-motion exercises, and

simple stretching regimens offer opportunities to socialize and can do wonders for your energy level, strength, and general feeling of well-being. Yoga and tai chi can help with balance, as well as providing a time for quiet meditation. Mindfulness classes can help you de-stress and focus on the most important things—your family and your life, rather than your illness. Your doctor or physical therapist can suggest an exercise program that will help keep you active no matter what your physical limitations or energy level. Ask several friends and/or family members to be your work-out buddies, so that you can have daily encouragement to adhere to your program.

Basic Concepts for People Who Help People with PD

17. **Go with the flow.** Periodically, the person with PD may experience hallucinations or delusions. It may be helpful to say, "I'm sure you really see the (little girl), but it's really the medication (or the Parkinson's disease) that's causing you to see (her). I'll call the doctor and see how we can make (her) disappear." Then redirect the person and say something

like, "Let's get a glass of ice tea. Come and help me." Or, explain that you're talking about what to get Mary for her birthday and ask, "What do you think she'd like?"**

18. **Be encouraging.** Whether it's getting the person with Parkinson's disease to exercise, eat, dress, or do any other activity, have a positive, patient, and encouraging attitude. Allow the person with PD to do as much for herself as possible. Squelch the tendency to jump up and do a task because you can do it faster and more easily than the person with PD. Encourage her to eat as much as possible independently before offering your assistance.**

19. **Expect the person with Parkinson's disease to participate in daily activities as much as he can.** Such activities such as setting the table, folding laundry, and putting groceries away keep one active and involved in everyday living.**

20. **Give verbal cues when necessary:** "Walk with me to the bedroom." Talk the person with Parkinson's disease through activities, like dressing and bathing. "Let's put on your shirt. Help me button your

shirt. Let's tuck in your shirt and button your pants." Be patient and encouraging to minimize the stress of the situation.**

21. **Encourage the person with Parkinson's disease to attend a support group meeting.** If that's not possible, try to arrange a one-on-one get together with another person with PD. If speech problems are not a factor, these "meetings" can be over the phone. Take care of yourself, too, and consider finding a caregivers' support group.**

22. **Contact the local fire department about any special needs the person with Parkinson's disease might have should a fire emergency occur.** The information will be noted and, in an emergency, the dispatcher will be able to tell the firefighters where to look for the person needing assistance (i.e., which apartment, which bedroom), and what special equipment or rescue procedures might be necessary. Communities vary as to how they record and retrieve this information; in some communities information between the fire, police, and emergency medical services is not shared. Even if your community has 911 emergency ser-

vices, you should contact your *local* fire department and emergency service agencies independently, *before* tragedy strikes.**

RESOURCES

Agencies, Organizations, and Web Sites to Help You and Your Family Learn About PD

American Parkinson's Disease Association, Inc.
1250 Hylan Boulevard, Suite 4B
Staten Island, NY10305-1946
800-223-2732
www.apdaparkinson.org

The Michael J. Fox Foundation for Parkinson's
 Research Grand Central Station
P.O. Box 4777
New York, NY10163
800-708-7644
www.michaeljfox.org

National Institute on Disability and
 Rehabilitation Research ABLEDATA
U.S. Department of Education
8630 Fenton Street, Suite 930
Silver Spring, MD20910
800-227-0216

www.abledata.com

The National Library Service for the Blind and
 Physically Handicapped
Library of Congress
Washington, DC20542
202-707-5100
TDD: 202-707-0744
www.loc.gov/nls

National Parkinson Foundation, Inc. Bob Hope
 Parkinson Research Center Bob Hope Road
1501 NW 9th Avenue
Miami, FL33136-1494
305-243-6666
800-327-4545
www.parkinson.org

National Rehabilitation Information Center
 (NARIC)
4200 Forbes Boulevard, Suite 202
Lanham, MD20706-4829
800-346-2742
TTY 301-459-5984
www.naric.com

Parkinson's Action Network
100 Vermont Avenue, NW, Suite 900
Washington, DC20005
800-850-4726

202-842-4726 or 202-842-4101
www.parkinsonsaction.org

Parkinson's Disease Foundation, Inc.
1359 Broadway, Suite 1509
New York, NY10018
800-457-6676
212-923-4700
www.pdf.org

Books and Newsletters

The Complete Directory for People with Disabilities, 2005 Edition
Grey House Publishing
185 Millerton Road
P.O. Box 860
Millerton, NY12546
800-562-2139
www.greyhouse.com/disabilities.htm

Demos Medical Publishing
386 Park Avenue South,
Suite 301 New York, NY10016
800-532-8663
www.demosmedpub.com

Disabilities Resources Monthly
Disability Resources, Inc.
Dept. IN

Four Glatter Lane
Centereach, NY11720-1032
631-585-0290
www.disabilityresources.org

Meeting Life's Challenges
9042 Aspen Grove Lane
Madison, WI53717-2700
608-824-0402
www.MeetingLifesChallenges.com

Resources for People with Disabilities and Chronic Conditions

Living with Low Vision: A Resource Guide for People with Sight Loss
Resources for Rehabilitation
22 Bonad Road
Winchester, MA01890
781-368-9094
www.rfr.org

Caregivers' Support Groups

Family Caregiver Alliance
180 Montgomery Street, Suite 1100
San Francisco, CA94104
800-445-8106

415-434-3388
www.caregiver.org

Independent Living Centers

National Council on Independent Living
1916 Wilson Boulevard,
Suite 209 Arlington, VA22201
877-525-3400
703-525-3406; TTY: 703-525-4153
www.ncil.org

Wheelchair Lifts

Bruno Independent Living Aids, Inc.
1780 Executive Drive
P.O. Box 84
Oconomowoc, WI53066
800-882-8183
262-567-4990
www.bruno.com

CHAPTER 2

Making Your Home Safe and Accessible

You can make many simple and inexpensive modifications to your home to make it more accessible without spending lots of money remodeling or making extensive changes. Associations that provide books, videos, and assistance in accessible home adaptations are listed in the Resources section at the end of this chapter.

23. **Some of the easiest changes you can make include the following:**

    • **Arrange furniture so that there are clear walking paths throughout the house.** Remove barriers such as magazine racks or footstools.

    • **Place furniture in strategic locations** in case you need to touch or hold onto it as you walk. Remove casters or wheels from furniture—objects that roll are an unstable means of support.

• **Remove throw rugs,** which may cause trips and falls.

• **Increase lighting** by using the highest wattage light bulbs recommended. Purchase a gooseneck lamp that allows you to adjust the lamp and shine the light in any direction.

• **Replace glass shower doors with a lightweight shower curtain** for easier access to the shower, greater safety, and convenience.

• **Store daily-use products like towels, dishes, food, spices, medications, and cleaning supplies between waist and eye level;** this will help you to avoid reaching and bending, which can throw you off balance and lead to falls.

• **Use reachers to relieve the strain of bending, stooping, or stretching.** Many different types of reachers are available; some models have pistol grips, others work like a giant pair of tongs, and some fold compactly to take with you.*

24. **Some people with PD propel them-selves forward when they walk, so that they have difficulty stopping quickly enough to avoid walking into furniture or through a glass door.** If this is a problem for the person you help, strategically arrange the furniture so you create soft landings, like the arm of an upholstered couch. *Note:* When considering this option, always consult the person with PD before rearranging any furniture, so that she does not lose familiarity with the surroundings.**

Lighting and Light Switches

25. **Replace traditional light switches with rocker-panel switches** that re-quire less fine motor control; they can be turned on or off by pressing with an arm, elbow, or palm of the hand. Some rocker panel switches are available with built-in illumination, so that you don't have to grope in a dark room to locate the switch. These are available at hardware and home-building supply stores.

26. **Purchase touch-sensitive lamps** if manipulating the small turn-screw on most lamps is difficult. Touch any metal on the lamp base and the light goes on; touch it a second time and the light goes off. If you use a three-way bulb, the light gets brighter with each successive touch, until the fourth touch turns it off. You can easily transform a traditional lamp into a touch-sensitive one by purchasing a converter kit. The converter screws into the receptor where the bulb normally goes; after you install a bulb, the lamp lights up when you touch it. Look for these at hardware and home stores.*

27. **Use TV remote to turn lights on and off.** Screw the Zapper Adapter into any light bulb socket and turn your light on and off with any regular, infrared remote control device. Install an adapter in one lamp in each room, carry the remote with you, and you will never be in the dark searching for the light switch again. The adapter has a 20-foot range with a lamp shade, 50-foot without, and will not interfere with the normal operation of the lamp. Maximum recommended wattage: 100 watts. Look for the Zapper

Adapter at hardware, discount, or numerous on-line stores.

28. **Install motion detector light switches** in the basement, garage, and utility room. Motion detector switches are especially useful in areas where you often find your arms full (with laundry, groceries, etc.). The light turns on when you enter the room and turns off a few minutes after you leave. You might also consider using photosensitive night-lights that automatically turn on at dusk.

Safety and Emergency Provisions

29. **Put glow-in-the-dark tape or stickers on the handles of flashlights** so that you can find them easily if your electricity goes out.

30. **If you have diminished sensitivity to temperature,** set your water heater's thermostat somewhere below 120°F to avoid accidental scalding while bathing or washing.

31. **Install smoke and carbon monoxide detectors** upstairs and downstairs in your home. Having smoke detectors is

important because the loss of the sense of smell is associated with Parkinson's disease. Having detectors for carbon monoxide, an odorless gas, is important in every home. Replace the batteries in these detectors once every year; replace the detectors themselves every 5 to 10 years.

32. **Use MotionPAD to alert you or others.** The Motion PAD is a motion sensitive device that chimes or plays a single prerecorded message when activated. Hang it on or place it near a door, and the chime will sound when the door is opened, signaling you that a confused adult is leaving the house. It also can be used to signal a care partner when assistance is needed, perhaps when medication wears off. Recording a message is easy and can be locked to prevent re-recording. Uses four AA batteries.*

33. **Driveway sensor gives advanced warning of visitors.** Install an electronic driveway sensor, and it will sound a chime and flash to alert you when a car approaches, giving you extra time to get to the door. The 1,000-foot range makes it perfect for long driveways. Some sensors

merely announce the arrival of a vehicle or person who crosses the path of their electronic beam. More advanced sensors have optional lamp controllers that, for added security at night or while you are on vacation, will turn on a light or radio, can be set to open a door or gate, or can be programmed to perform different functions based on whether a car is arriving or departing.*

Doors, Doorways, and Doorknobs

34. **Replace regular doorknobs with lever handles** or purchase a rubber lever that fits over any standard doorknob. Lever handles are easier to operate—just push down with your hand, arm, or elbow. Purchase lever handles at hardware or home building supply stores. You can make a doorknob easier to grasp by wrapping several rubber bands around the largest part of the doorknob to increase its diameter.

35. **Create extra wheelchair clearance in doorways.** You will need a minimum of 32 inches of clearance to get the average wheelchair through a doorway. To make

your home doorways more wheelchair accessible:

• Cut out the doorjamb molding starting from the floor and going up 3 to 4 feet. Removing this portion of the doorjamb will add an extra 1 1/2 inches clearance for the wheelchair to get through and still allow the door to function normally.

• For a temporary solution, you may simply remove the molding altogether, understanding that the door will not latch or have the stop guard that the molding provides.

• Another option is to install offset hinges that allow the door to swing out and away from the doorway opening, increasing the door opening 2 to 3 inches. For a source of offset hinges see the Resource section of this chapter or speak to a hospital occupational or physical therapist.*

36. **Door stop sign or mural camouflages dangerous attractions.** If your loved one gets confused and wanders into dangerous places, placing a stop sign or photographic mural on tempting doorways may help keep them safe. A large red stop sign (10 1/4 inches square) sends

an understandable message not to exit through a doorway or enter "off limit" rooms. The sign mounts directly to the door with Velcro strips (included); it wipes clean with soap and water. A photographic mural looking like a set of bookshelves camouflages doorways to stairs and storage closets, effectively making them "disappear." The 3-foot 2-inch by 8-foot 8-inch mural comes in two pieces for easy installation using double-faced tape (included). Please note: These items are no substitute for locks on doors leading to dangerous areas.*,**

Under Lock and Key

37. **Buy adaptive key devices that fit on regular keys and give better leverage for turning.** Hardware, home health care, medical supply stores, and catalogs have different styles; be sure to try them first to see which works the best for you.

38. **Keep a full set of duplicate keys in several places around the house,** in case you misplace a set. Always try to put the keys you regularly use in one designated place (say, in a dish or on a hook by the door most frequently used)

to reduce the amount of time you spend hunting for them.

39. **Install a keyless entry system.** A wireless, remote door entry system allows access to your home without traditional keys. A battery-powered key fob remotely activates the lock from up to 164 feet away, even while an occupant remains seated or in bed. The lock system can be mounted to any wooden door, operates cylinder and night-latch locks, and can be used in conjunction with traditional key locks for added security. For maximum security, the easy-to-program and re-program fobs use a "rolling code" that changes each time the door is released. The entry system comes with two key fobs, but up to ten can be added. It requires a 12-volt plug-in power supply.*

40. **Install a doorbell/intercom system.** Someone with PD may not be able to get to the door before a visitor leaves. No one wants to miss an important delivery or visit, especially if the visitor doesn't know to wait for you. This problem can be surmounted with a special doorbell/intercom system that is easily installed in most homes by a qualified electrician. The

system works like this: When a visitor rings the doorbell, every telephone in the house starts to ring (even cordless phones). When you answer the telephone, it works like an intercom so that you can communicate with the person waiting outside. If you are on the phone when a visitor arrives, a call waiting tone will sound to alert you. If you have a second doorbell at a side or back entrance to your house, the system can be wired with a distinct telephone ring for each doorbell. Some advanced systems even allow you to unlock the door from your telephone.*

Ramps, Railings, Stairs, and Grab Bars

41. **If the person with PD uses a wheelchair, install a ramp with a railing.** Be sure there is a level area in front of the door; a platform 5 feet wide and 3 feet long is recommended at the top of the ramp to allow room to unlock and open the door. Railing height above ramps is a matter of personal preference. The average-sized person usually finds a height of 35 to 36 inches works well; if the person using the wheelchair is short, consider one that is 32 to 34 inches high.

Railings, 1 1/4 inches to 1 1/2 inches in diameter, should be installed on both sides of the ramp and placed so that 1 1/2 inches of clearance is available from any obstruction such as a wall.**

42. **Install hand railings on both sides of a stairway** wherever you have stairs, both inside and outside the house, even if there are only one or two steps, as on a front porch. Handrails on both sides give the dominant grip a firm hold both going up and down stairs.

43. **Consider installing a railing along a long hallway in your home.** That way, if you need to steady yourself or rest, you have additional support.

44. **Place U-shaped handles strategically near doorways** to help you navigate through the doorways more easily. If you tend to fall backward when opening a drawer, door, or cabinet, you may want to install U-shaped handles nearby to help you keep your balance.

45. **Install grab bars wherever you need to hold onto something sturdy,** espe-

cially when transferring from one place to another, such as to the toilet or tub. Decide where the grab bars will provide you with the most help, and leave a space the width of a clenched fist (about 1 1/2 inches) between the grab bar and the wall. Vinyl-covered grab rails are better for grip and will absorb less heat in exterior locations.

46. **When installing railings, U-shaped handles, or grab bars that will be used to support your weight, make sure they are securely anchored to the studs in the wall.** Get professional advice on proper placement or hire a professional if you are unable to do the installation yourself.

47. **Install a support pole by the bed, toilet, living room chair, and dining room table.** You can use these poles to steady yourself, as a balancing aid, and to help you get to a standing position.*

• The Guardian Safe-T-Pole is held in place by controlled tension and requires no special tools or structural changes for installation.

• The Super Pole System is a modular support system that provides assistance with standing, transferring, or moving in bed; this floor-to-ceiling pole is installed by a simple jackscrew expansion.

• The Advantage Rail is a portable model that can be taken with you or moved out of the way when not needed. It quickly secures and releases from a low-profile, floor-mounted plate; additional floor plates can be purchased to use the pole in multiple locations.

48. **Install a stairlift for people who have difficulty navigating stairs.** You might want to consider installing a stair lift if you have difficulty getting up and down stairs because of limited mobility, tremors, poor eyesight, or wheelchair use. These devices, which are installed on the wall of your stairway, allow a person to sit on a chair at the top or the bottom of the stairs and be glided to the opposite end by the power lift.*

The Kitchen

49. **If you plan to purchase new appliances,** consider buying a stove with a

smooth top; it is much easier to clean. Select a side-by-side refrigerator/freezer, so that you can store both frozen and refrigerated items at eye level.

50. **Store dishes, utensils, and food in locations closest to where you use them.**

• Store dishes and glasses over the dishwasher or sink; hang pots and pans from hooks near the stove; and keep frequently used items on the countertop or in another convenient location.

• Avoid stacking or piling objects on top of each other.

• Label the drawers, cupboards, and cabinets in the kitchen with a description or a photo of the contents. This cuts down on the amount of time spent searching for items, especially if others frequently help you in the kitchen.

• Place commonly used items on a turntable or lazy Susan in the center of the kitchen table or on a countertop. You might also use a lazy Susan in a deep cabinet or cupboard, so that you can access the contents more easily.

51. **Look for a cutting board with a raised side** or have wooden sides attached to your existing cutting board to minimize spilling diced food. Boards with stainless steel prongs help hold foods in place while you cut.*

52. **Purchase a dustpan attached to a long handle** so that you won't have to bend over. You can collect your floor sweepings while in a standing position. You might also try using a child's broom from a sitting position.

53. **Use Pow-R-Grips handles with brooms and other long-handled tools to improve leverage and help reduce wrist and back strain, blisters, fatigue, and repetitive stress injuries.** Made of durable nylon plastic, each set of Pow-R-Grips handles consist of two pieces that are used together—the straight grip handle is placed on the upper portion of the long-handled tool, while the D-grip handle is placed at the mid-point of the tool. Pow-R-Grips are sold in sets of one

straight grip handle and one D-grip handle.*

The Bathroom

54. **Crisscross two pieces of adhesive tape over the bolt on the bathroom door.** Adults who are confused or have trouble operating a doorknob will not be able to lock themselves in the bathroom.**

55. **If the bathroom doorway is too narrow to manage, remove the door** and replace it with a tension rod and an opaque or black shower curtain liner. This will provide more clearance, helpful not just for wheelchair users but also for those who use a walker or require assistance.

56. **Purchase a telescoping mirror** that either clamps to the side wall of the vanity or sits on top of the vanity counter. Telescoping mirrors feature adjustable, swivel-type necks that can be moved to various positions easily. Usually, one side has a regular mirror and the other a magnifying mirror, making it perfect for makeup application and shaving. Another option is

to install mirrored tiles at various heights on the bathroom walls.

57. **If you have separate controls for hot and cold water, consider installing wrist blades.** Wrist blades are wide, wing-type handles that can be operated by pushing with the forearm, wrist, or heel of the hand. These are available at most plumbing supply and hardware stores.

58. **Install kitchen faucets in bathrooms.** To make it easier to get your hands under the water, you may want to replace bathroom faucets with kitchen faucets, which are longer and project farther into the sink basin.

59. **Install an automatic faucet that turns water on and off automatically.** Some models turn on with slight pressure on a wand and turn off when pressure is released; others are activated by an electric eye.*

60. **Purchase an inexpensive resin or webbed outdoor chair or bench so that you can sit while bathing or showering.** This will reduce your risk of

slipping in the shower. Purchase these chairs at home supply or discount stores.

61. **Consider buying a removable shower-head.** on a flexible, hand-held extension hose. They are fairly inexpensive, easy to install, and make showering much easier, especially if you're sitting on a tub bench or shower chair. However, a hand-held shower nozzle can be very slippery and hard to grip when your hands are soapy; you'll have better control if you wind several rubber bands around the handle portion of the nozzle. You will find hand-held showerheads at hardware or home stores.

62. **A bath lift or bathtub transfer bench can make getting in and out of the tub much easier.** Bath lifts connect to a faucet or shower pipe and use water pressure to lower you into and raise you out of the water; they have hand controls, so that you can operate them without assistance. Some models are portable and lightweight, so that you can take them with you when you travel. Ask an occupational therapist about how to set up and adjust an appropriate bathtub transfer bench.*

63. **Purchase an adjustable portable toilet seat.** to increase the height 3 to 7 inches and make it easier to get on and off the toilet. Some raised seats provide armrests for added support; all easily attach to any toilet. Models that come with a lock are the safest, because the lock prevents the seat from slipping off the toilet during a transfer. Buy a tote bag so that you can take the seat with you and safely use bathrooms away from home, too.

64. **Consider purchasing an uplifting commode** that assists you in rising from the toilet.*

The Bedroom

Setting Up the Bedroom

65. **The bed should be low enough for you to get in and out easily.** A good guideline is for the bed to be 22 inches high, but take your height into account. In general, if the bed is lower than knee height (like a futon), getting in and out will be difficult. If your bed is too low, set its legs on recessed wooden risers (blocks with holes cut into them to accom-

modate the bed legs). If your bed is too high, consult a carpenter to get the legs of the bed shortened.

66. **If nighttime incontinence creates occasional problems,** buy a plastic mattress cover at a discount store or a waterproof pad at a store where cribs or baby products are sold. The waterproof pad is a flat piece of flannel-like material that sits on the mattress in the middle of the bed. Place the pad under the fitted sheet or make the bed with two fitted sheets, placing a waterproof pad between the sheets. If the top sheet gets wet, remove it and the pad, and you have a clean bed in a flash.

• If nighttime incontinence problems are chronic, consider wearing adult incontinence briefs.

• Be sure to discuss any incontinence problems with your doctor or a specialist.

67. **If the person with PD spends lots of time in bed, make the bedroom a pleasant place to be for both of you.** Orient the bed so that it faces a window. Bring in fresh flowers. Hang a frame or

bulletin board with pictures of family and friends where it can easily be seen.**

68. **Try a vibrating pillow to relieve stiff, tight, or achy muscles.** The pillow is designed to strap onto a headboard, the back of an office chair, or car seat. Remove the detachable strap, and you can position the pillow to massage your neck, back, shoulders, legs, and feet. Because the pillow vibrates quietly, you won't disturb others if you use the pillow in bed or during a meeting. Manufactured by Health Solutions, the pillow, which requires 4 AA batteries, is available at Walgreen Drug Stores.

69. **Keep a water container with lid and drinking straw by the bedside.** Many sports bottles or children's cups come with a built-in fold-down straw. These drink containers are also good for travel, because they won't spill if tipped over.

70. **Hang shoes by their laces or straps over the handle of your closet door,** so that you won't trip over them. In addition, you won't have to bend over to pick up the shoes.

Bed Rails and Bed Pulls

71. **Consider repositioning your bed against the wall** to make it more accessible. Install a grab bar on the wall alongside the bed, about 10 inches higher than the mattress. Be sure to anchor the railing to studs in the wall so that it will be secure. Another option is half bed rails that can be installed under the mattress. Installing such rails might eliminate the need for an expensive hospital bed with bed railings.*

72. **Attach a bed pull to the grab bar or to the frame at the foot of your bed** to assist in turning over and getting out of bed. Use a nylon rope, or braid three pieces of tightly woven fabric together, in a length that will reach from the base of the bed to your hand when lying down. It should be long enough for you to reach, but still at arm's length for good leverage when you want to pull yourself out of bed. Tie a large wooden ring to the end to serve as a handhold. Then sew a binder clip (butterfly clip) near the ring, so that the bed pull can be clamped to the bedding and remain within your reach. You may want to at-

tach another bed pull to the side of the bed to assist you in turning.

Turning Over in Bed

73. **Use satin bed sheets.** Their slippery surface makes it easier to turn over in bed. Flannel sheets make it more difficult to turn over than standard cotton or percale sheets.

74. **Consider installing a trapeze or harness that hangs over the bed,** so that you can grab hold of it to lift and turn yourself.

75. **Place a long, sturdy cardboard box under the covers at the foot of the bed.** Elevating the covers will keep pressure off your feet and legs and allow you to turn without getting tangled up in the bedding.

76. **If you need to move or reposition someone with Parkinson's disease in bed,** here is a technique you can use:

    • Create a draw sheet by placing a flat sheet, folded to fit from the person's chest to the thighs, over the fitted sheet on the bed. This is what you'll use for leverage underneath the person.

• Grab the sheet with your palms up, count to three, and move/pull the person and draw sheet toward you.

• To do a two-person lift to reposition the person up or down in the bed, count to three and shift your body weight from the back to the front leg, keeping your arms and back in a locked position. Move in unison to slide the person.**

77. **Use baby monitors to hear a person with PD who is in bed.** The monitor's transmitter sits on the bedside table and the receiver goes in another room for remote listening. Some monitors have portable receivers, so that you can listen to the person as you move around the house.**

78. **Help the person with PD feel relaxed in the bedroom** by implementing a few of these tips:

• Give the person a back or leg massage.

• Keep a favorite blanket or pillow on the bed for comfort and security. Don't purchase new linens without checking to see if the person with PD likes them. Bringing unfamiliar items into the environment can be very upsetting to people with PD, especially those who are confused or have dementia.

• Use a night-light or leave the bathroom or hall light on to help keep the person with PD oriented to where she is.**

Furniture and Floor Coverings

79. **Walking or wheeling on carpet is easier if the carpet pile is very short.** It is easier still on wood, linoleum, or ceramic floors; however, bare floors and ceramic tiles can be slippery when wet, so use caution. You may want to consider changing the floor covering or surface.

80. **Use furniture that is sturdy and stable.** Generally, the best sitting chair has a relatively straight back, a firm, shallow seat, and armrests. Avoid low, heavily upholstered couches and chairs, because it is often difficult to rise from them without help. Sofas or chairs should be

approximately 17 inches off the ground; the seat should be no lower than knee height. Add a firm cushion or attach risers to the chair legs to increase the height of the chair. For some, a comfortable, heavy rocking chair with armrests may help, because it can give you an extra boost when rising.

81. **Place a clear plastic chair protector on upholstered dining room chairs** and gain several advantages—prevents spills from staining fabric and makes it easier to change position and slide on and off the chair seat.*

82. **To get out of a chair,** scoot forward to the edge of the seat, spread your feet apart, and rock back and forth to build up momentum.

RESOURCES

Home Accessibility Ideas and Environmental/Home Adaptations

Adapting the Home for the Physically Challenged
(Video) A/V Health Services, Inc.
P.O. Box 1622

West Sacramento, CA95691
703-389-4339

Consumer's Guide to Home Adaptation
Adaptive Environments
374 Congress Street,
Suite 301 Boston, MA02210
617-695-1225 (V/TTY)
www.adaptiveenvironments.org

National Kitchen & Bath Association
 (Barrier-Free Planning)
687 Willow Grove Street
Hackettstown, NJ07840
800-843-6522
877-NKBA-PRO
www.nkba.org

Helpful Products for People with PD

Automatic Faucet
Ageless Design, Inc.
12633159th Court
North Jupiter, FL33478-6669
800-752-3238
www.alzstore.com

Bath Lifts, Benches, and Seats

Bruce Medical Supply
411 Waverly Oaks Road, Suite 154
Waltham, MA02452
800-225-8446
www.brucemedical.com

Sammons Preston Rolyan
An AbilityOne Company
270 Remington Boulevard, Suite C
Bolingbrook, IL60440-3593
Worldwide Telephone: 630-226-1300
TDD 800-325-1745
www.sammonspreston.com

Sunrise Medical (North American Operations)
7477 East Dry Creek Parkway
Longmont, CO80503
800-333-4000
303-218-4500
www.sunrisemedical.com

Bed Rails

Bed Handles
4825 South Tierney Drive
Independence, MO64055
800-725-6903
www.bedhandles.com

Access with Ease
P.O. Box 1150
Chino Valley, AZ86323-1150
800-531-9479
928-636-9469
www.shop.store.yahoo.com/capability/

Easy Street
509 Birchwood Court
Raymore, MO64083
800-959-EASY (3279)
www.easystreetco.com

Sammons Preston Rolyan
An AbilityOne Company
270 Remington Boulevard,
Suite C Bolingbrook, IL60440-3593
Worldwide Telephone: 630-226-1300
TDD 800-325-1745
www.sammonspreston.com

Driveway Sensor

Smarthome
16542 Millikan Avenue
Irvine, CA92606
800-242-7329
www.Smarthome.com

Doorbell Intercom System

Smarthome
16542 Millikan Avenue
Irvine, CA92606
800-242 7329
www.Smarthome.com

Door Stop Sign/Mural

Ageless Design, Inc.
12633159th Court North
Jupiter, FL33478-6669
800-752-3238
www.alzstore.com

Keyless Entry System

Eazykey Ltd.
202 Three Elms Road
Hereford, UK HR4 0RF
011-44-0870 046 0878
www.eazykey.com

MotionPAD

Attainment Company, Inc.
504 Commerce Parkway
P.O. Box 930160
Verona, WI53593-0160

800-327-4269
www.attainmentcompany.com

Offset Hinges

Dynamic Living
428 Hayden Station Road
Windsor, CT06095-1302
888-940-0605
www.dynamic-living.com

Plastic Chair Protectors

Solutions Catalog
P.O. Box 6878
Portland, OR97228-6878
877-718-7901
www.SolutionsCatalog.com

Pow-R-Grips Handles

Total Living Company
5 East Napa Street
Sonoma, CA95476
707-939-3900
www.totalliving.com

Reachers

Access with Ease

P.O. Box 1150
Chino Valley, AZ86323-1150
Orders: 800-531-9479
928-636-9469
www.shop.store.yahoo.com/capability

Specialty Cutting Boards

Active Forever
10799 North 90th Street
Scottsdale, AZ85260
800-377-8033
www.activeforever.com

Life with Ease
P.O. Box 302
Newbury, NH03255
800-966-5119
www.lifewithease.com

Stair Lifts

Bruno Independent Living Aids, Inc.
1780 Executive Drive
P.O. Box 84
Oconomowoc, WI53066
800-882-8183
262-567-4990
www.bruno.com

Support Poles

Advantage Rail
Health Craft Products, Inc.
2790 Fenton Road
Ottawa, Ontario, CANADA
K1T 3T7
888-619-9992
613-822-1885
www.healthcraftproducts.com

Guardian Safe-T-Pole

Sunrise Medical (North American Operations)
7477 East Dry Creek Parkway
Longmont, CO80503
800-333-4000
303-218-4500
www.sunrisemedical.com

The SuperPole System

Health Craft Products, Inc.
2790 Fenton Road
Ottawa, ON, Canada
K1T 3T7 888-619-9992
613-822-1885
www.healthcraftproducts.com

Touch-Sensitive Lamp Converter

Products for Seniors
850 South Boulder Highway,
Suite 171
Henderson, NV89015
800-566-6561
www.ProductsforSeniors.com

Uplift Commode

Easy Street Co.
509 Birchwood Court
Raymore, MO64083
800-959-EASY (3279)
www.easystreetco.com

CHAPTER 3

Looking Good, Feeling Better

When you look good, you tend to feel better. In this chapter, you'll find ways to streamline dressing so that you'll have more time and energy to pursue other daily activities. But first, here are some basic concepts to keep in mind:

- Dressing will be easier when your medications are working, so plan to dress during your "on" time.

- Allow enough time so that you don't feel rushed. Gathering all your clothing items together before you start to dress will save steps and time. You may even find it helpful to lay your clothes out the night before. Then, if you plan to wear something that requires assistance (i.e., hooked at the back) you can ask for help before family members go off for the day.

- If your balance is unsteady, sit on the bed or in a sturdy chair with armrests when you dress. You may also want to sit when you do your hair, shave, or apply makeup.

Grooming

83. **Substitute a wash mitt or soft sponge for the usual washcloth.** A wash mitt slips on the hand and can be easier to use than a washcloth. A sponge or lightweight cotton dishcloth is lighter and easier to wring than terry cloth washcloths. A long-handled sponge or bath brush can be used to reach your legs, feet, and back without bending.

84. **Use soap-on-a-rope** to prevent the slips and falls that can occur in the shower when you bend to retrieve a dropped bar of soap. Hang the soap around your neck or within easy reach over the shower nozzle.

If you can't find soap-on-a-rope at the drug store, make your own. Cut the leg from an old pair of pantyhose; place a bar of soap in the foot area; securely tie the top thigh area of the hose to the pipe behind the showerhead; then stretch the hose and lather up. Another option is to use shower gel on a bath pouf or sponge instead of a bar soap.

85. **Pour shampoo onto a sponge;** then rub the sponge on your hair. The shampoo is less likely to run into your eyes, and there's no chance of dropping a slippery bottle in the tub or shower.

86. **Keep several sets of clean undergarments in a drawer** in the bathroom so that you can change into them after you shower.

87. **Cut your toenails right after you bathe,** since they are less brittle and will be easier to cut. A toenail clipper or pair of scissors with short blades works best. However, if your nails are too thick, select a heavy-duty pair of scissors or consider having your toenails cut by a pedicurist or podiatrist.

88. **After eating, cleanse your mouth of any residual food** and rinse with antibacterial mouthwash. Maintaining good oral hygiene is especially important because of the swallowing problems often associated with PD that can leave food in your mouth that attracts harmful bacteria that not only affects your oral health but can damage your heart as well.

89. **Use an electric toothbrush.** If you have tremors, brushing your teeth thoroughly with a traditional toothbrush can be difficult. Some electric models have long, easily grasped handles, some are cordless, and some feature dual motion (up and down, side to side). If you prefer the manual method, try using a toothbrush with an oversized handle, available at most drug stores. Whichever method you choose, conserve energy by brushing your teeth while sitting down and resting your elbow on the bathroom counter.

90. **Buy dental floss "swords"** that look like the letter "C," with floss stretched tight across, at the end of a plastic toothpick. Available in drug stores and grocery stores, they let you floss with one hand. The water action of a Water-Pik will massage your gums and rinse food debris from your mouth. (It takes some dexterity to use a WaterPik, so if you have tremors, you might want to stick to rinsing with a sip of water or mouthwash and using dental floss "swords.") You can get electric flossers as well. Check your local pharmacy for options.*

91. **Consider purchasing Toothettes,** a sponge coated in dried toothpaste, attached to the end of a small stick. They're great for cleaning out the mouth and getting to those areas a toothbrush can't. When brushing isn't convenient, dampen it with water or dip it in a little mouthwash to clean out your mouth.

92. **An Oral Care Kit provides instruction and tools to help facilitate brushing someone else's teeth.** The kit consists of a package of four Open Wide Disposable Mouth Rests, one Surround Toothbrush, and an instructional video entitled "How to Brush the Teeth of Another Person."*,**

93. **Use an electric razor if you experience tremors.** Electric razors come in many shapes, some of which are easier to hold than others. Test out how they feel in your hand before you buy one.

94. **Use pump-type containers for lotions and liquid soap.** It's often easier to press down on a pump top than to squeeze a bottle or grasp a bar of soap.

95. **Easy Reach Lotion Applicator helps apply lotion to hard to reach areas.** This completely washable device features a long, curved plastic handle and a soft, nonabsorbent pad that allows you to apply creams, lotions, or sunscreens to those hard-to-reach places on your back and body without help from others. It's ideal for people whose ability to reach or bend is limited.*

96. **Use a countertop hair dryer.** If holding or aiming a hair dryer is difficult, try a countertop dryer stand that has a stable base and moveable neck. Insert your blow dryer handle into the cushioned holder at the top and, to dry your hair, simply turn your head in front of the stream of air.*

Choosing the Right Clothing

97. **Take the hassle out of finding the right clothing.** If shopping for new clothes is overly taxing, call your favorite clothing store and schedule a convenient time when a sales clerk can give you individual attention. In some cities, stores offer personal shopping services; a personal shopper will listen

to your clothing needs and specifications and find the appropriate items for you. You can also order from retailers with catalogs or web sites if you prefer to shop from home.

98. **Replace clothes that are hard to put on with easy-on/easy-off clothing.** You may want to buy clothing one size larger than you normally wear.

99. **Choose satin or nylon tricot sleep-wear.** Turning over in bed will be easier because of the slippery surface of satin.

100. **Choose underwear made of nylon** instead of cotton. You will have an easier time pulling slacks and trousers up and down.

101. **Choose clothing that closes in the front if you dress yourself.** If your arms are stiff, and you need help dressing, purchase or make shirts that open in the back but look like front-opening shirts.*

102. **Choose shirts with multiple colors and patterns.** If you tend to spill when eating, most spills won't show up.

103. **Look sharp with pre-knotted ties.** If you have difficulty tying a necktie, try adjustable, pre-knotted zipper ties. Zipper ties are worn by putting the loop over the head, under the shirt collar, and then pulling downward to adjust the fit. They come in a variety of colors and are perfect for dressy occasions, because they look neat and tidy—much harder to detect than clip-on ties.*

104. **Choose clothing with elastic waistbands or Velcro closures** instead of zippers or buttons. Sweatpants that are made of double-knit fabric and have elasticized waistbands generally are easier to put on and take off. Wear pullover tops to eliminate fastening.

105. **Choose a roomy, easy-to-put-on robe.** Change-A-Robe is a hooded, poncho-style robe made of thick quality velour terry cloth that is roomy, easy to put on, and has large pouch pockets to store tissues, glasses, reading material, even a change of clothing. The unisex robe features a full hood, deep scoop neck, one large inside pouch (which can be accessed from inside or outside the robe), two large outside pockets, and a

zippered front opening. This robe is everything in one—dry off with it, wear it to stay warm, change under it, or use it as a blanket. One size fits all. For people in wheelchairs, the Handi-Robe is designed to be put on without having to stand.*

106. **Purchase swimsuits that wrap around the body** and are extremely easy to put on and take off.*

Dressing Tips

107. **Always dress a weaker limb or your stiffer side first.** To undress, take the garment off the stronger side first.

108. **To remove a shirt or blouse,** unbutton the garment and ease it off your shoulders. Reach behind your back and gently tug the garment off.

109. **Dress in front of a mirror.** It will help you find the sleeves and match up buttons and buttonholes. Button garments from the bottom up, so that you're less likely to skip a button. Or, button the bottom few buttons and put the garment on over your head.

110. **If you're wearing layers,** such as a turtleneck underneath a sweater, put the turtleneck inside the sweater before dressing (don't forget to pull the sleeves through) so that you will only have to expend the effort of putting the garments on one time.

111. **If the person with Parkinson's disease is easily confused or upset by change,** try to always dress him in the same type of clothing (e.g., sweatpants, a short-sleeved shirt, and a zip-front cardigan).**

Dressing Aids and Simple Clothing Adaptations

112. **Use Velcro to replace buttons and other fasteners.** Sew an existing buttonhole closed and sew a button on top of it. Then, sew the soft fuzzy side of the Velcro on the underside of the closed-up buttonhole. Sew the other piece of Velcro, the hard side with the small hooks, where the button used to be.

113. **Sew buttons on with elastic thread.** If buttoned cuff openings are too small

to pass your fist through, move the buttons to make the opening larger and/or sew the buttons on with elastic thread. The elastic thread will give the rebuttoned cuff opening an extra quarter inch or so.

114. **Make your own zipper pull** by screwing a small cup hook into a dowel. Use it to zip up jackets and dresses. If your fine motor coordination is impaired, a buttonhook handle is easier to grasp than a small button. A buttonhook slips through the buttonhole and pulls the button back through it. Buttonhook handles come in various sizes and finishes (wood, rubber, etc.).

115. **Use a dressing stick** so that you can dress while seated (thus reducing your risk of falling). A dressing stick is a long stick with a hook or clamp on the end that you can use to grab items of clothing or accessories and position them on yourself without straining, bending, or reaching. The dressing stick will also help you to reach clothing or shoes that have fallen to the floor.

116. **Sew loops of bias tape inside the waistbands** of slacks and trousers. Use the loops to pull pants up and down.

117. **If a waistband is too tight, extend it** by putting a covered ponytail band or rubber band through the buttonhole and wrapping both loops around the button.

For commercial sources for dressing aids, see the Resources section at the end of the chapter.*

Hosiery and Footwear

118. **Choose the right shoes.** If you have a shuffling gait, soft rubber soles make walking more difficult, especially on carpeting, where the soles can stick and cause you to trip. Hard leather soles can be very slippery on linoleum or tile floors.

119. **Use elastic shoelaces** in place of normal laces, so that you will only have to tie your shoes once. Just slip your shoes on and off.*

120. **Have a shoemaker convert your traditional tie- or buckle-close shoes into Velcro-closing shoes.** Or buy slip-on shoes instead of tie shoes.

121. **Put on your shoes with a long-handled shoehorn** to minimize bending and reaching.

122. **Wear tube socks.** Tube socks are easier to put on than socks that are shaped like a foot. Sew loops into the inside of each sock and use the loops to pull on your socks.

123. **Support hose and compression socks may relieve painful, swollen feet.** Support hose, available at travel shops and pharmacies, give your legs extra support for less fatigue and better circulation. Compression socks must be prescribed by your doctor; your insurance might cover part or all of the cost. Putting on the socks requires some strength and practice, and you may need assistance. The socks come in navy, black, and flesh tones.*

124. **Sprinkle cornstarch on the bottom of your feet** and around the heel area

to make pulling on nylon stockings or socks easier.

125. **Alter your slacks to accommodate an ankle-foot orthotic (AFO) brace.** If you wear an ankle-foot brace that fits inside a shoe and goes up the calf, it will be easier to dress if you sew a 7-inch zipper into the inside seam of your slacks.

RESOURCES

Adaptive Clothing

Adaptations by Adrian
P.O. Box 7
San Marcos, CA92079-0007
877-6-ADRIAN (23-7426)

American Health Care Apparel, Ltd.
302 Town Center
Boulevard Easton, PA18040
800-252-0584
www.clothesforseniors.com

Buck & Buck
311127th Avenue, South
Seattle, WA98144
800-458-0600

Epiphany Design
84 Carlton Street,
Suite 904 Toronto,
Ontario M5B 2P4
Canada
888-410-2243
416-410-2243
www.epiphanydesign.ca

AutoFlosser

DDS Products, LLC
23852 Pacific Coast Highway,
Suite 788 Malibu, CA90265
800-200-5553
www.autoflosser.com

Change-A-Robe

Creative Designs
3704 Carlisle Court
Modesto, CA95356
800-335-4852
209-523-3166
www.robes4you.com

Dressing Aids

Access with Ease
P.O. Box 1150

Chino Valley, AZ86323-1150
Orders: 800-531-9479
928-636-9469
www.shop.store.yahoo.com/capability

Independent Living Aids, Inc.
200 Robbins Lane
Jericho, NY11753-2341
800-537-2118
516-752-3135
www.independentliving.com

Sammons Preston Rolyan An AbilityOne
 Company
270 Remington Boulevard,
Suite C
Bolingbrook, IL60440-3593
Worldwide Telephone: 630-226-1300
TDD 800-325-1745
www.sammonspreston.com

Elastic Shoelaces

Zackaroos
Steven Enterprises
6053 Third Avenue
South Minneapolis, MN55419
612-869-9794
www.zackaroos.com

Hair Styling Stand

Active Forever
10799 North 90th Street
Scottsdale, AZ85260
1-800-377-8033
www.activeforever.com

Latex-Free Swimwear

Suits Me Swimwear
5114 Menominee Line Road
Gillett, WI54124
352-666-1485
www.latexfreeswimwear.com

Lotion Applicator

Easy Street Co.
509 Birchwood Court
Raymore, MO64083
800-959-EASY (3279)
www.easystreetco.com

Oral Care Kit

Specialized Care Co.
206 Woodland Road
Hampton, NH03842-1542
603-926-0071

800-722-7375
www.specializedcare.com

Support Hose and Compression Socks

Jobst USA
www.jobst-usa.com

MediUSA
P.O. Box 3000
Whitsett, NC27377-3000
800-633-6334
www.mediusa.com

TravelSox
The Summit South,
Suite 450S
300 Centerville Road
Warwick, Rhode Island 02886
866-387-6762

Zipper Ties

Silvert's
3280 Steeles Avenue West, Suite 18
Concord, ONL4K 2Y2
Canada
800-387-7088
905-738-4545

72

www.silverts.com

CHAPTER 4

Communicating

Parkinson's disease (PD) can affect communication in many ways. Your ability to speak can diminish because of the disease itself or because of the medications used to control your symptoms. It is important, though, that you talk for yourself whenever possible. Don't get into the habit of letting others do all the talking for you. Have a discussion with your family and friends about your speech problems, and let them know ways they can help you. Encourage them to ask you to speak louder or ask for a repetition. Try not to be defensive when asked to repeat yourself. Staying calm will make it much easier for you to be heard and understood. If you are frustrated when a well-meaning family member attempts to fill in words when you pause in a sentence, let her know that you just need a little more time to finish and that you'd appreciate the chance to speak on your own. Set some ground rules about which approaches to communication work for you and which approaches you find less helpful. *The important thing is not to let speech difficulties prevent you from communicating and participating in social activities.*

People with PD sometimes experience the loss of facial expression (masked faces) and have a fixed stare. When this happens, many non-verbal cues are lost and misunderstandings and miscommunications can occur. For example, a person with PD may look bored or disapproving, which may not be the case at all. If your facial movements lack expression, make an extra effort to express verbally how you feel and what you are thinking.

Your handwriting may also be affected by PD. Many people find that their writing grows smaller and smaller with each word or letter (micrographia). You might be inclined to give up writing. Don't! Writing is a form of exercise for your hands and arms, and continuing to use those muscles will maintain their condition. Try printing instead of writing in cursive, it can be more legible.

This chapter discusses additional tips for improving your ability to communicate.

Speaking Tips

126. **Take time to organize your thoughts and plan what you are going to say.** If you have trouble remembering or pronouncing a particular

word, think of a related word to get your idea across.

127. **Take a breath before you start to speak** and pause every few words, or even between each word. Learn to use your diaphragm when you breathe. (Your stomach will move up and down rather than in and out.) When you breathe correctly, it will to help improve the volume at which you speak, and you will have enough air to finish a sentence.

128. **Face your listener.** It will be easier for you to communicate if you can both see each other's faces and if you have each other's full attention. Don't try to carry on a conversation with someone who is in a different room or whom you can't see.

129. **Have conversations in a quiet environment,** so that you can hear and be heard better. This is especially important if your voice is soft or you have trouble hearing.

130. **Swallow any excess saliva before you attempt to speak.** If dry mouth

is a problem, keep a water bottle handy, so that you can take a sip before speaking.

131. Use shorter sentences or use only the necessary words to get the message across, even if it's not in complete sentence form.

132. **Exaggerate your pronunciation of words.** Force your tongue, lips, and jaw to work hard as you speak. Enunciate as if your listener is hard of hearing and needs to read your lips. Finish saying the final consonant of a word before beginning the next word. Precise word endings are necessary to determine word meanings (e.g., *them* versus *then*).

133. **Make a conscious effort to vary your facial expressions** to reflect your mood and the message you're trying to convey. Sometimes, with PD, your face is less expressive than it used to be. Integrate the following warm-up activities into your morning or evening washing ritual:

• Massage your facial muscles.

• Practice in the mirror. Open and close your mouth; alternate smiling and pursing your lips; raise and lower the tip of your tongue, then move your whole tongue from side to side.

• Consciously raise your head to an upright position. Think about how your head and neck feel.

• Try some verbal warm-ups, like reciting a poem or singing a song.

134. **If you find you are easily distracted while talking, close your eyes.** This will minimize environmental distractions and reduce the pressure you feel in watching the other person waiting for your next word. If you are talking while walking, pause for a moment before closing your eyes (Remember to open your eyes again before you resume walking!).

135. **Use gestures while you talk** to make yourself understood. If you can't think of the word, try pointing to an object you are discussing.

136. **If possible, write what you want to say** or use a communication board featuring words, the alphabet, or pictures.

137. **When you are frustrated, count to ten.** Allowing stress and frustration to get the better of you will make it even harder for you to communicate.

138. **Use these word-finding tips** if you can't think of the word you want to say:

• Say the first sound of the word a few times until the rest of the word comes to you, or say a word that rhymes with the one you want. Ask the person you're speaking with to help come up with possibilities until you get to the right word.

• Go through the alphabet in your head until you come to the letter with which the word begins.

• Use a category approach: If you are trying to remember the word for a new item of clothing you bought, think of the words for other kinds of clothing. (Think,

"Jacket, slacks, socks, shoes..." until you get to "sweater.")

139. **If you find yourself having unusual difficulty finishing a conversation,** take a break and return to the conversation after you've had a chance to rest a bit.

140. **Have your hearing and the hearing of the person with PD checked** to keep your communication from being adversely affected by an inability to hear each other.**

141. **Hold conversations at eye level** and make eye contact during conversation. Sit down if the person with PD is sitting, and assume a relaxed posture to convey your patience and willingness to listen. Speak clearly and calmly and allow enough time for a thorough exchange of words. Be patient—most people with PD who have difficulty speaking have no cognitive difficulty (meaning their minds are just fine); instead, their muscles and nerves are preventing them from speaking as clearly as they did in the past.**

142. **Avoid finishing sentences for someone with PD** unless he asks for your help finding a word or phrase. Reinforce instances of good, intelligible speech. Give feedback such as a nod of the head or a "yes" or "I see" to indicate that you understand what he is saying. However, don't say you understand when you really do not. Repeat any part of the message you did understand and ask for clarification or repetition of the rest. Asking for a repetition of a phrase can result in clearer pronunciation the second time around.**

143. **Ask the person with PD to restate a phrase or sentence using different words.** If you cannot understand what was said, ask for clarification; if you pretend to understand to save time, misunderstandings can result. In addition, the person with PD may not make as much of an effort to speak clearly if she thinks you understand.**

144. **Ask questions that require yes/no answers.** For example, instead of asking, "What would you like to eat?" ask, "Would you like a turkey sandwich?" Or, ask questions that will elicit one-word,

or short-phrased responses. Ask, "What kind of meat would you like on your sandwich?" instead of "What do you want for lunch?" Or, offer a few choices when you ask a question: "Would you like soup or a sandwich for lunch? Would you like tomato soup or chicken noodle soup?" Use some gentle prompts before beginning a new topic of conversation. Say, for example, "Let's talk about your grandchildren." When you change the subject, use similar cues ("Let's talk about the Super Bowl now").**

145. **Give verbal cues before assisting someone with Parkinson's disease.** If you're going to help someone with an activity, tell the person what you are about to do before you touch him. This will reduce your chances of startling the person. For example, before guiding the person to the door, say, "Let's goes outside now."**

Using Technology to Aid in Spoken Communication

146. **Speech amplifiers can be helpful to people with PD who have a weak voice,** throat, or chest muscles, partially

paralyzed vocal cords, or diminished lung capacity. Speech amplifiers are like portable public address systems; they can improve one-on-one and group communication by allowing the speaker to use her normal tone, yet amplified so that listeners can hear the voice better. Some amplifiers are pocket size and some have handheld or headset microphones.*

147. **Use communication tools.** Go Talk is an easy-to-use, portable communication tool that allows the user to call for help or make simple requests with the touch of a button. It records up to 36 messages (9 message keys with 4 distinct levels) for a total of 6 minutes recording time. A record lock eliminates accidental erasures, a level-lock option prevents unintentional level changes, and built-in-key guards help users select the right message. It is easily programmable in any language, and it operates on two AA batteries (included).

Another way to make communication easier is by using picture cards depicting common words, items, phrases. Make your own or purchase ready-made sets in a variety of topics.*

148. **Replace hard-to-use telephones** with models that are easier to use and actually enhance your ability to communicate:

• Make a cordless phone even easier to use by adding a headset, which looks like a headband with a microphone and earphone. Clip the phone to your belt or set it in your lap, and then you can talk hands-free. Headsets cost about $20 and are sold wherever phones are sold.

• Use big-button telephones with large buttons and raised or enlarged numbers and letters. Giant pushbutton telephone adapters slip easily over the face-plate of most touch tone phones, and they double the size of the numbers to make them easier to see and press.

• Look for telephones with a volume control in the receiver, so that you can easily turn the volume up or down during a call.

• Use the special features available on many phones today. Hands-free speaker-phones, with built-in speakers and automatic dialing, can be fitted with headsets and special on/off switches. Speakerphones and cordless phones often have intercom capabilities, which can be particularly helpful for communicating with people in other rooms of the house.

• Learn how to program your telephone's auto-dial or speed-dial function to eliminate the need to dial frequently used numbers. If that is too difficult, have a friend or family member program the phone for you and explain how to use the speed-dial features. Write directions down on an index card and keep the card next to the phone or tape the instructions onto the handset of a cordless phone so that they are always there when you need them.

• Use pictures to help you remember who to call. Seeing a picture can be a better memory jogger than if just names or phone numbers are written on the phone. Place up to eight pictures of family and friends in the Memory Phone, program the corresponding telephone numbers into the phone and, with just the push of a "picture," place your call. If you prefer, tape small photos of each person next to the speed dial buttons for friends and family on your existing telephone.*

149. **An Automatic Telephone "Hanger-Upper" keeps loved ones in touch.** For families worried about the forgetfulness of a loved one who lives alone or far away, the Automatic Telephone "Hanger-Upper" (3 by 4 by 1 1/8-inches) may be a solution. This device disconnects the phone line so that the phone will still ring, even if the person forgets to place the handset back into the cradle. The device plugs into a wall outlet (adapter included) and works in conjunction with your existing telephone.*,**

150. **A dial-less telephone eliminates inappropriate calls.** If your loved one calls over and over or throughout the night, the dial-less telephone may bring relief. This telephone looks like a regular phone, yet has no numbers to dial. Your loved one can receive calls, but not call out. *Recommended only for those living in residences where alternative measures are available for real emergencies.**,**

151. **Make sure you have at least one "hard-wired" phone in case of emergency.** When the power goes out, cordless phones, which rely on electric power to operate, will not function. Make sure you have at least one "hardwired" or "land-line" telephone that will continue to function if the power is out. A cell phone is also good to have in case of emergencies.

Writing Tips

152. **Keep your hand and arm muscles in the habit of writing by taking up drawing or painting.** Not only will you improve the condition of your muscles, but you may find a new artistic talent. If you don't want to start with a blank page, purchase coloring books that have designs, costumes, and nature scenes to color.

153. **Try writing with the hand you don't normally use.** Practicing this can keep both sides of your brain active.

154. **Try printing letters in the opposite direction of what you usually do.**

For instance, if you normally write the letter P starting with a straight down-ward stroke and then lift your pen to add the half-circle to the top, try starting at the bottom of the P and, without lifting the pen, add the half-circle in one continuous stroke. Or, make the half-circle first and add the stick later.

155. **Buy pens and pencils with wide grips (at least 1 1/2 inches or 3 cm), because they are easy to grasp and use.** Make holding a standard pen or pencil easier by trying one of the following:

• **Twist a rubber band several times around a pen or pencil.** Roll it into position where your fingers rest. The rubber band will widen the barrel and help you keep your grip.

• **Slip a 2-inch piece of rubber tubing over the barrel of a pen or pencil** to make the grip easier to use.

• **Use pen or pencil grips.** These grips are small, cylindrical pieces of rubber with a hole in the center. The pen or pencil fits through the hole, and you adjust the rubber grip until it is in a comfortable writing position. It stays in place until you move it or take it off. These devices can be found at office or school supply stores.

156. **Bring along several preprinted, self-adhesive address labels** (with your name and address) when you attend conventions, forums, store openings, or any other place where you might need to fill out forms. Instead of writing all your information on the form, use your address labels when you want to sign up, register for prizes, or send away for information. You can also purchase a rubber stamp with your address or signature on it.

Keeping the Lines of Communication Open

157. **Use the computer to communicate when speaking or writing is too difficult.** Going online and communicating with others will help keep your mind active. Using e-mail can be a wonderful way to keep in touch with family and friends.

158. **Use Speech-to-Speech Relay (or Telecommunications Relay Service).** This federally mandated service is for people whose speech may be difficult to understand because of a medical condition or because they use a voice synthesizer, voice enhancer, or electrolarynx. The service helps remove the communication barriers that people with speech disorders face when they are doing something as basic as ordering a pizza or making a doctor's appointment. The person with the speech disability calls the telecommunications relay system in his state and a specially trained communication assistant (CA) takes down the number that the person with the speech disability wants to call, places the call, and acts as an interpreter for the conversation. For example, to make a doctor's appointment, the CA calls the doctor's appointment desk on the phone, listens to the person with the speech disability, and repeats the message word-for-word to the doctor's receptionist. Communication continues with the CA acting as the voice of the person with the speech disorder.

The telecommunications relay system also facilitates calls between people who use a standard phone and those who use a TTY (or text telephone) due to hearing impairments. As of March 1, 2001, all states are required to provide Speech-to-Speech/Telecommunication Relay Services 24 hours a day, 7 days a week. Check the "Rights and Responsibilities" pages in the opening pages of your local telephone book, or call your state's Department of Administration for details.*

159. **Contact your library for information** about firms handling specialized communication equipment and the names of associations and support groups.

160. **Encourage friends and relatives to each choose a specific time each day or each week to call.** Having short (2- or 3-minute) conversations on a regular basis can go a long way toward helping the person feel included and loved, especially if she can't get out socially.**

161. **If someone you care for is unable to leave home for special events,**

such as reunions and weddings, use a video camera to document the event. Have people at the event record special greetings for the person who was unable to make it. If you move to a new home, and your loved one cannot visit, make home videos of your new house, the neighborhood, the kids' school, soccer field, library, and other places you frequent and might talk about. When you deliver the video, give a running narration of the scenes shown on the screen. It can be a great way to spend time together and keep the person involved in your life.**

162. **Use your camcorder to create a video "card" for someone who can't get out to visit family and friends.** Record well-wishes and other greetings and take footage of some of the person's favorite places. This unique document will spark fond memories and show the person that he is remembered.**

RESOURCES

Communication Tools for Speech and Language Impairments

Attainment Company, Inc.
504 Commerce Parkway
P.O. Box 930160
Verona, WI53593-0160
800-327-4269
www.attainmentcompany.com

Dial-less Telephone

Ageless Design, Inc.
12633159th Court
North Jupiter, FL33478-6669
800-752-3238
561-745-0210
www.alzstore.com

Memory Phone

Ageless Design, Inc.
12633159th Court
North Jupiter, FL33478-6669
800-752-3238
561-745-0210
www.alzstore.com

Speech Amplifiers

Amplivox Sound Systems
3149 MacArthur Boulevard
Northbrook, IL60062
847-498-6691
orders: 800-267-5489
www.ampli.com

Chattervox
847-816-8580
www.chattervox.com

Luminaud, Inc.
8688 Tyler Boulevard
Mentor, OH44060
800-255-3408
440-255-9082
www.luminaud.com

Park Surgical Co., Inc.
5001 New Utrecht Avenue
Brooklyn, NY11219
800-633-7878
718-436-9200
www.parksurgical.com

Speech-to-Speech Relay

STSnews

P.O. Box 100607
Milwaukee WI53210
www.stsnews.com

Telephone Hanger-Upper

Ageless Design, Inc.
12633159th Court
North Jupiter, FL33478-6669
800-752-3238
561-745-0210
www.alzstore.com

CHAPTER 5

Managing Mealtime Madness

The kitchen is often the busiest room in the house. It becomes a hotbed of activity when you're preparing and eating meals. The chapter on General Home Accessibility shares kitchen organization tips; this chapter will help you plan, make, and serve meals so that you can streamline the process and make tasks easier.

Begin by building more time into your schedule to prepare and eat meals. Make the kitchen or dining room a calm, low-stress environment by playing soft, relaxing music while you cook and eat.

Do as much planning and preparation as possible while seated at the kitchen table or at a stool pulled up to a countertop. If your energy or medication's effectiveness waxes and wanes, prepare meals when your energy level is high, and reheat and serve food after you've had a chance to rest. When eating, sit close to the table and place all food and utensils within easy reach.

In the Kitchen

Meal Planning and Preparation

163. **Choose a grocery store that will not defeat you before you begin.** When deciding on a store, take into account not only prices and location but also layout and facilities, including restrooms. Is the store accessible? Are the doors easy to manage? Are the floors clear of debris and obstacles?

164. **Ask if your neighborhood grocery store has a home delivery service,** if getting out to shop for groceries is a problem. Some stores will charge a flat fee, while others will require a minimum order. Delivery areas vary, and so does how far in advance you must call to place your order. Large chain stores or warehouse-type grocery stores rarely deliver, but they often have the names and phone numbers of delivery services that do.

165. **Online grocery stores are a convenient way to shop.** To avoid going out in inclement weather, you can periodically place your order over the Internet or

schedule the regular delivery of your favorite foods. Unfortunately, this type of service only covers certain areas of the country. Continue to check these web sites for changes in their delivery areas. Also, check your local grocery stores to see if they offer online grocery shopping or home delivery.*

166. **If you don't want to walk unassisted through a slippery parking lot,** some grocery stores will send a bagger or stock person to help you get from your car to the store and back again. Other stores may allow you to pull up to the front door and have an employee park your car. These services usually are available to regular customers who have made arrangements in advance. Another option is to park next to the area where shopping carts are kept outside. Pushing a shopping cart can improve your stability when walking through the parking lot and store.

167. **Ask the bagger not to fill your bags too full.** Spread out the items into more, but lighter-weight, bags. Ask that all frozen or perishable foods be put into one bag. Then, when you arrive home,

you only need to empty one bag immediately; the others can wait.

168. create a diagram of the store and list the food categories for each aisle. Then, make a master list on your computer of items you buy. Before you go to the store, print out a list and circle each item you need. This method is especially helpful if you send a friend to do your grocery shopping—there is no question about what brand and what size of a particular item you want.

169. **Use a wagon (like a Radio Flyer) or a wheeled wire cart to move groceries from the car to the house.**

170. **Meals on Wheels is a national organization that provides prepared meals to your door,** usually by volunteers through local senior citizen centers and organizations. For homebound seniors or their care partners who have a limited ability to acquire meals by traditional means, Golden Cuisine delivers nutritious frozen meals, weekly, anywhere

in the United States. Specifically designed for seniors by registered nutritionists, meals range in price from $3.70 to $4.70, with a $7.50 shipping charge per seven-meal package. Golden Cuisine meals can be ordered via the Internet through CareGuide (www.careguide.com) or Meals on Wheels Association of America (www.mowaa.org). Check with your local United Way agency for availability.*

171. **Encourage the person with PD to be involved in activities like sorting things**—putting away groceries, setting the table, and putting away clean silverware and dishes. If items are not put in the proper spot, quietly move them to where they belong.**

172. **Improve your grip to open a jar by:**

• Putting on a rubber glove,

• Winding a thick rubber band twice around the lid, or

• Using a 5 by 5-inch, thin, waffle-grid rubber sheet. These rubberized sheets, available where kitchen gadgets are sold, make untwisting caps and lids easier.

• Using a jar opener that attaches to the underside of a cabinet.*

173.	**Use a rocker knife instead of a traditional straight knife.** You can get a seesaw motion going with the rocker knife and use less energy than that required with a straight knife.

174.	**Keep an extra pair of pliers in the kitchen.** Use them to peel away the plastic seal from a jar of peanut butter, to pull the tab on a container of cream cheese, or to grab the sealer strip from a can of frozen orange juice or a gallon of milk.

175.	**To get an easier grip on cooking tools, replace old kitchen gadgets and utensils with modern gadgets that have large, cushioned handle grips.** Many discount, housewares, and grocery stores carry a wide selection of potato peelers, spatulas, whisks, and more. OXO International offers a complete selection of specialty and hard-to-find cooking utensils (cookie scoop, spice grinders) and other easy-grip products and tools for your home and garden.

176. **Angled measuring cups let you read measurement markings by looking straight down into the cup, eliminating the need to tip your head to check the amount of liquid you are measuring.** The soft, nonslip handle provides a firm grip; cup, ounce, and milliliter measurement markings increase convenience. Available in 1–, 2–, and 4–cup versions, the measuring cups are dishwasher safe. You will find them at discount and department stores.

177. **The Prep Taxi safely carries food from cutting board to pan or bowl.** This unique scoop allows you to slice, dice, and chop food in preparation for cooking and, with one easy motion, safely transfer it to your cooking pan or bowl. Its flat design, 6-inch wide mouth and 1-inch high sides, contains food to prevent spills. Made of rustproof 18/8 stainless steel, the scoop holds up to 3 cups.*

178. **Purchase jelly in plastic squeeze bottles,** so that spreading it on sandwiches is easier.

179. **If you have tremors, prepare finger foods that don't require the use of a knife and fork.** Purchase cheese cubes, precut chicken strips, and cocktail-sized hot dogs just to name a few. In the produce section of the grocery store, you'll find cut-up fruits and vegetables. While they sometimes cost more than the uncut variety, the time and energy you save can be worth every penny.

Making and/or Using Simple Adaptive Devices at Mealtimes

180. **If grasping and holding onto silverware is difficult,** use modeling clay; foam tubing, which comes in a variety of thicknesses; or heat-activated pellets to build up the handles on utensils.*

Another solution is to purchase stainless steel flatware with big bamboo or plastic handles that are easier to grip. Some specialty catalogs and medical supply stores sell inexpensive utensils specially designed for easy use.*

Note: Using weighted, built-up utensils may also help decrease tremors while eating.

181. **Use a glass or metal pie pan instead of a regular plate,** if you have trouble keeping food from sliding off the plate. Use a plate guard or a pasta bowl with high sides, because it will be easier to get food onto the spoon or fork. Plate guards can be attached to plates to provide a rim on one side. Use your fork to push food against the guard, where food will fall onto the fork. Plate guards also help reduce spills.*

182. **Place Dycem rubber pads or Rubber-maid mats underneath plates, cups, and serving dishes** to keep them from sliding.*

183. **If you have hand tremors or a weakened grip, make handling a drinking glass an easier task with these suggestions:**

   • Fill glasses half-full.

   • Wind several thick rubber bands around the glass.

• Drink from a plastic water bottle (or sports bottle) instead of a glass. The small opening at the top prevents beverages from sloshing out; when sealed, the cap prevents spills if the bottle is accidentally bumped or tipped.

• Use a flexible plastic drinking straw instead of drinking directly out of a glass. To better hold a straw in place, find a lid of a plastic container (the same diameter as your glass), punch a hole in the lid, and insert a straw into the hole. You'll find that the straw does not slide around in the glass.

• Use a child's cup with a built-in straw for drinking. The Tommee Tippee cup is made of unbreakable plastic and has a spout and a see-through cover. The curved base is weighted to prevent spilling.

• Drink from a cup or mug that has two handles.*

184. **Protect your clothes when eating with a Gourmet Guard napkin.** If hand tremors make it difficult to eat without spilling, a moisture-proof, dis-

posable napkin from Gourmet Guard may help. These large napkins have an adhesive strip along the top that sticks to your clothes; they can be used as a bib or lap napkin.*

Eating and Drinking Tips for People with Swallowing Difficulties

Swallowing is a very complex process, and difficulties in chewing or swallowing (dysphagia) can cause additional health problems. It is estimated that 50 percent of people with PD will experience dysphagia at some time during the course of their illness.

If you experience difficulty swallowing, ask your doctor for a referral to a speech/language pathologist (SLP), along with a prescription for "swallowing evaluation and therapy." A swallowing study and a video fluoroscopic evaluation by a specially trained SLP can best diagnose exactly what part of the swallowing process is causing you problems and recommend a treatment program for you. You and the people who help you will learn important tips that can help keep you healthy.

One important consideration affecting swallowing ease may be when you take your medication. Consult with your physician on how to time your medications to facilitate swallowing and experiment with what works best for you.

To Reduce Swallowing Difficulties

185. **Plan a regular mealtime schedule.** Give yourself at least twice the time it usually takes to eat a meal. Don't allow yourself to feel hurried, because stress can exacerbate symptoms and make swallowing even more difficult. Minimize mealtime distractions by turning off the television and radio and keeping conversation to a minimum. To keep your food warm for a longer period of time, consider using a child's heated plate.*

If you find that you fatigue quickly when eating a whole meal, plan five or six smaller meals during the day, or snack throughout the day. If chewing is too difficult, but your swallowing is good, drink a food supplement such as Ensure, Boost, or Carnation Instant Breakfast to supplement your diet. Check with your doctor to make sure that the protein content of those drinks doesn't interfere with the absorption of your medications. You might also consider juices or smoothies made from fresh ingredients.

186. **Suck on a few crushed ice cubes about 20 minutes before mealtime** to reduce any swelling in your throat. If you eat something very cold and sour, like lemon or lime sorbet, before you begin to eat, it may help to improve saliva production for people with dry mouth; it may also stimulate the muscles necessary for swallowing and reduce tongue delay. Although not proven, it may be helpful to eat spoonfuls of the cold, sour food periodically during the meal to continue improved swallowing and to help clear the mouth and throat of food particles.

187. **Sit in an upright position with both feet on the floor** and stay upright for at least 30 minutes after a meal. Reclining or lying flat while eating can cause food to remain in the esophagus or to back up into it. If you have frequent heartburn, it is important to consult with a good gastroenterologist. Frequent bouts of heartburn can damage the esophagus. In rare cases, food can be refluxed all the way up and into the

throat. The major danger when that happens is that some of the refluxed material could get into the airway and down into the lungs. When foreign material gets into the lungs, it can cause pneumonia.

188. **Keep your chin pointed down as you chew and swallow.** In addition, gently touching or massaging the front of the throat right before or during eating may help stimulate swallowing.

189. **Concentrate on each step of the swallowing process.** Make sure you have enough saliva or moisture in your mouth to get the food into your esophagus. Do not try to eat if you are too fatigued to concentrate on chewing and swallowing.

190. **Take bite-sized portions** (about one-half spoonful) of food. Chew deliberately. Swallow each bite completely before you take another. Chew hard with the food on one side of the mouth, then move the food to the other side and chew hard some more. Take comfortable sips of liquids to reduce the risk of aspiration. If swallowing liquids at the same time

as solid foods is difficult, stick to one substance at a time before you try to swallow another.

191. **If you have a cough that you can't stop,** try eating a spoonful of applesauce. Its cool, smooth texture can help soothe your irritated throat. Applesauce now comes in single-serving cups, so you can carry one with you for instant relief.

However, if your cough persists, food may have gone down into your airway. A cough is your body's natural protective mechanism for getting rid of foreign material in the airway. The signs of silent aspiration (food particles that go into the airway but you do not feel them) may be respiratory problems, fever, chest noises, and then pneumonia. Consult a doctor immediately if you experience any of these symptoms.

192. **If you feel that you are choking while swallowing,** close your mouth, breathe through your nose, and calm down. Taking that one breath will give you enough air to help avoid panic and allow you to breathe normally again. Ask family members and helpers to learn the Heimlich maneuver in case you choke

while trying to swallow. A doctor or other healthcare professional can demonstrate and teach the procedure.

Tips If Drooling Is a Problem

193. **When drooling is a problem, chew gum.** It helps remind you to swallow more often.

194. **Make it a deliberate habit to try to swallow your saliva regularly.** To reduce its accumulation in your mouth, close your lips firmly, move the saliva to the back of your throat, and swallow. Swallow any excess saliva before you attempt to speak.

Food Consistency and Texture

195. **The texture of food becomes more important when** you can taste only sweet, sour, or salt. See which textures work better for you. However, if you have trouble swallowing, be sure to have a swallowing study done, which can tell you if thickened liquids might help and how to experiment with various degrees of thickness.

196. **Swallowing can be easier if you stick with foods of a soft, even consistency.** An example would be creamy, whipped mashed potatoes (not lumpy and dry or thin and runny, but smooth and somewhat viscous, like sour cream).

197. **Avoid foods that easily pose a choking hazard:**

• Steak is the number one thing people choke on. Eat ground steak instead.

• Dry foods that break into small pieces like seeds, nuts, or baked goods.

• Foods that irritate your throat (such as vinegar) or cause you to choke (potato chips, etc.).

198. **Stick with foods that are easy to swallow:**

• Baby foods and cereals. Baby foods have a smooth, easy-to-swallow consistency.

• Strained, thickened soups. Puree a favorite soup in a food processor or blender to remove chunks. Then, thicken the soup with mashed potatoes (or strained, mashed peas, beans, lentils, or chick-peas), blend, and serve.

• Strained, thickened fruits. Use a food processor to combine your favorite fruits with cottage cheese, cream cheese, or yogurt. Strain off excess liquid, blend until desired consistency is reached, and then serve.

• Yogurt. Buy the smooth or blended variety, or puree the fruit-on-the-bottom variety in a blender until smooth.

• Thick puddings.

• Soft bread with crusts removed. Take your time with bread. Eat one small piece at a time. Suck on it until it is soaked in saliva and swallow it with one big gulp.

• Canned liquid diets. Some of these may be too thin; thicken them with corn-starch. Be aware that relying solely on liquid diets can result in low blood albu-min, so you might want to add dried egg-white powder to the liquid if you plan to use liquid diets for an extended period.

• Fruit nectars. Thicker than most juices, nectars are less likely to be aspirated when swallowed. Look for apricot, pear, mango, and banana nectar in the ethnic or specialty aisle of your supermarket. Tomato juice is another thicker beverage that can be easier to swallow.

• Thick spreads like hummus or cream cheese. Serve on soft, crustless bread or eat as a snack with a spoon.

• Mashed avocado or banana.

199. **Try variations on your favorite food and drinks** to make them easier to swallow. For example, if you find regular orange juice irritating to your throat, try orange juice with pulp or the low-acidity kind.

Swallowing Pills and Vitamins

200. **Some pills can be difficult to swallow;** ask your doctor or pharmacist if your medication will retain its potency if it is ground up and com-

bined with food. If your doctor advises against grinding up your pills, try swallowing the pill with fruit nectar instead of water. Try swallowing it along with a spoonful of applesauce or honey, or coating the pill with a little butter or pudding.

201. **Put the pill into your mouth, tilt your chin down, look down into the bottom of your glass of water, and swallow.** Continue to look down during the entire swallowing process. Some people find that this works much better than tilting your head backward when swallowing a pill.

202. **Thickeners can make liquids and prepared foods easier to swallow.** Food thickeners can be mixed with liquids and prepared foods to thicken them to whatever consistency you desire. Several brands are available.*

203. **"Swallowing Safely, Swallowing Nutritiously: A Manual for the Swallowing Impaired"** written by Maxine Dereiko, a registered, licensed dietitian and Patricia Stout M.S., C.C.C. and "Recipes for Easy Chewing and Safe

Swallowing" by Dereiko and Elaine Teutsch, R.N., M.S. offer help to people with moderate to severe swallowing problems. $12.50 plus $7.50 for shipping and handling. Allow 4 to 6 weeks for delivery.*

204. **Many adaptive devices make meal preparation, eating, and drinking easier.** See the Resources section for a list of companies with a wide product selection.*

RESOURCES

Adaptive Products

Easy Street
509 Birchwood Court
Raymore, MO64083
800-959-EASY (800-959-3279)
www.easystreetco.com

Maxi Aids, Inc.
42 Executive Boulevard
Farmingdale, NY11735
Information: 631-752-0521
TTY 631-752-0738
To order: 800-522-6294
TTY 800-281-3555

www.maxiaids.com

Sammons Preston Rolyan
An AbilityOne Company
270 Remington Boulevard, Suite C
Bolingbrook, IL60440-3593
Worldwide Telephone: 630-226-1300
TDD 800-325-1745
www.sammonspreston.com

Automatic Jar Opener

Active Forever
10799 North 90th Street
Scottsdale, AZ85260-6726
800-377-8033
www.activeforever.com

Drinking Cups and Mugs

Sammons Preston Rolyan
An AbilityOne Company
270 Remington Boulevard,
Suite C Bolingbrook, IL60440-3593
Worldwide Telephone: 630-226-1300
TDD 800-325-1745
www.sammonspreston.com

Dycem

Dycem Limited 83
Gilbane Street
Warwick Central Industrial
Park Warwick, RI02886
800-458-0060
www.dycem.com

Food Thickeners

Bruce Medical
411 Waverly Oaks Road, Suite 154 Waltham,
 MA02452
800-225-8446
781-894-6262
www.brucemedical.com

D.C. Distributors, Inc.
P.O. Box 224
Amherst, NY14226
800-827-6763
716-825-5834
www.dcdistributors.com

Med-Diet Laboratories
3600 Holly Lane, Suite 80
Plymouth, MN55447
800-MED-DIET (3438)
www.med-diet.com

Gourmet Guard Napkin

AgeNet, Inc.
17 Applegate Court;
Suite 200
Madison, WI53713
Phone: 888-405-4242
www.agenet.agenet.com

Heated Plate

Maddak, Inc.
661 Route 23 South
Wayne, NJ07470
973-628-7600
www.maddak.com

Inner-Lip Plate

Maddak, Inc.
661 Route 23 South
Wayne, NJ07470
973-628-7600
www.maddak.com

Meal Delivery Services

Golden Cuisine
Kitchens of ConAgra Foods
6 ConAgra Drive

PDL-375
Omaha, NE68102
800-886-4084
www.goldencuisinestore.com

Meals on Wheels
National Office
1414 Prince Street,
Suite 302 Alexandria, VA22314
703-548-5558
www.mowaa.org

On-line Grocery Services

www.homegrocer.com

www.netgrocer.com

www.peapod.com
800-573-2763

Prep Taxi

Solutions Catalog
P.O. Box 6878
Portland, OR97228-6878
877-718-7901
www.SolutionsCatalog.com

Swallowing Books

Dereiko-Teutsch & Associates
P.O. Box 8366
Portland, OR97207
503-241-8077
www.dereiko.com

Swivel-Tremor Spoon

Maddak, Inc.
661 Route 23 South
Wayne, NJ07470
973-628-7600
www.maddak.com

Thermo Pellets

North Coast Medical, Inc.
18305 Sutter Boulevard
Morgan Hill, CA95037-2845
800-235-7054
www.beabletodo.com

CHAPTER 6

Empowering Yourself

Life is about choices. You may not have total control over your Parkinson's disease (PD), but you *do* have control over how you let it affect your life. Staying active and involved is possible with effort and determination.

Keep moving. Eliminate distractions, and tell your family and friends that you may not be able to carry on a conversation while you are walking. If crowds or long-distance walking is involved, use a cane or walker for stability. Pushing a baby stroller or shopping cart may can help you maintain balance. Using a wheelchair may be a good option, especially at museums, sidewalk art shows, and amusement parks. Choose to make the necessary compromises and adjustments, so that you can stay involved in family and community activities.

Another way to stay active and involved is to continue doing the quiet leisure activities you enjoy. If the effects of PD or your medications make your favorite hobby difficult to pursue, try a variation on your hobby or learn a new craft. Keep your mind and your hands active by doing jigsaw puzzles, taking up painting or woodworking, or playing a musical instrument. Take a class, so that you can learn along with others and meet new people who share your interests. You'll socialize and learn something at the same time. If you have a skill that you haven't used in a while, pick up a beginner's book at the library and refresh your memory with introductory lessons. You'll be surprised at how quickly you can relearn a skill you thought you'd forgotten. Don't be hard on yourself if it takes you a while to master a new craft. Everybody has a learning curve; don't let initial frustrations discourage you from keeping at it.

Some people who have PD have trouble with concentration, memory, or communication. If you feel these abilities have been affected, help is available. Discuss your concerns with your doctor, and ask to see a psychologist who will be able to help you identify exactly what cognitive deficits you might be experiencing and help you develop plans to keep effectively on track.

Here are some other tips to get you moving, involved, and enjoying the fun things in life.

Mobility and Exercise

Walking

205. **Walking with someone can be better than using a walker.** Hold onto the arm of someone else while walking, and say out loud together, "Left, right, left, right, left, right." This might help you concentrate on your movements. Your physical therapist (PT) can help determine when using a walker is safer.

206. **When walking, bring your toes up with every step you take.** If you tend to shuffle, follow these steps:

   • Stop walking.

   • Make sure your feet are about 8 inches apart. • Stand up as straight as you can.

   • Think about taking a large step.

   • Take a step by bringing one foot up high, as if you are marching.

- Lift your toes up and place your heel down first.

- Roll onto the ball of your foot and toes.

- Repeat this process with the other foot.

- Swing your opposite arm forward when taking a step. This will improve the rhythm of your walking and your appearance. Swinging your arms freely while walking shifts body weight from your legs, lessens fatigue, and helps loosen your arms and shoulders.

207. **If you drag your foot, see an orthopedic specialist.** Untreated, your foot dragging will become worse, and you will trip yourself. Your orthopedist can make arrangements for you to get an ankle-foot orthotic (AFO) brace. If stumbling persists, see your neurologist.

208. **When you want to turn, walk into your turn.** Walk around in a semicircle with your feet apart; don't pivot on one foot by crossing your leg.

209. **Try marking your floors with a grid** of 18-inch squares of colored electrical

tape. Some people with PD find that it is easier to walk in the squares of tile flooring.

210. **Ask first, "Would you like help?"** Never grab an arm or try to help a person without permission. Let the person with PD tell you how to help her. Remember, you are supplying balance control not physical support. Don't try to pull the person along or lift her.**

211. **Before you start walking, count down** from the number five to the number one and on one, begin walking. Let the person whom you are assisting set the pace. When appropriate, announce upcoming changes in the terrain ("There's a step down.")**

212. **To help a person with PD walk, stand in front of him and hold his hands.** When you walk backwards, gently guide him forward. Give verbal cues like "Let's walk now."**

213. **If the person with PD wears bifocals, he may need extra help when using stairs.** Going down stairs is often more difficult than walking up. When we go

upstairs, we usually look through the top (or long-distance range) part of the lens, but when we go downstairs, we look down (through the near-distance or reading part of the lens). Looking down, our feet aren't close enough for our eyes to focus on through the reading part of the bifocal. No matter which direction you are going—up or down stairs—watch carefully.**

214. **When assisting someone walking up or down stairs, take one stair at a time.** Let the person you are assisting hold onto a handrail, if one is available. Make sure she places each foot completely on each stair. When going up stairs, have the person lead with the stronger foot. When going down stairs, have the person lead with the weaker foot. Stand in front of the person when descending stairs, and behind the person when ascending the stairs.**

Tremors

215. **If you have a tremor, wait until it stops to resume your move-**

ment. Tremors often decrease when you stretch your hands and arms out in front of you.

216. **If a resting tremor interferes with activities involving your hands,** press the affected elbow against your body to stabilize the upper arm, and then perform the desired movement as quickly as you can.

217. **Wear exercise weights around your wrist** (known as wrist weights) to help stabilize and reduce the frequency and duration of tremors.

Freezing

218. **To get "unstuck" from a freeze that may occur when you approach narrow spaces,** try these tips:

   • Don't try to take any steps.

   • Place your heels on the floor.

   • Straighten yourself into an upright posture; don't lean backward or forward.

• Gently rock side to side.

• Take a few marching steps in place.

• Start taking steps forward by placing your heels down first.

• Keep your feet about eight inches apart and correct your posture as you go.

219. **If you freeze when walking,** try these tips:

• Very carefully walk backward or sideways.

• Count from one to ten, or count by twos to twenty, with the idea in mind that you'll walk when you reach the last number.

• Ask your helper to gently rock back and forth with you to get you moving.

• Try dancing instead of walking. Whistling or singing may also help you overcome freezing.

• Focusing on the beam of a flashlight or laser pointer may break a frozen gait. Use a credit card-type flashlight instead of a bulky wand-style flashlight. The credit card varieties are lightweight, convenient, and activated with a gentle squeeze. Some come with a key chain attached, which you can hang from a bedpost, wheelchair, or walker.

• Try lifting just your toes.

• Have someone drop pieces of a tissue on the floor like stepping stones and use them to break your freeze.

220. **Using a cane can help with freezing.** If you use a cane with a small golf club-type protrusion at the bottom, it can make walking easier because it tricks your mind into thinking you're stepping over something.

221. **Take a collapsible cane with you when you walk.** When you freeze, assemble the cane and gently kick the end near the floor.

222. **When you can't walk a step forward,** take a small step *back,* then

rock forward and go. When you can't turn left, take a small step *right,* then rock to your left foot and go.

223.   **When the person with PD gets stuck in a freeze,** try taking his hands in yours (as you face him) and gently pumping your hands up and down in an alternating motion.**

Standing Up, Sitting Down

224.   **If you have trouble standing up from a seated position,** try these techniques:

• Put your hands on the armrests, rock back and forth, and count.

• Ask someone to stand in front of you and wiggle or dance.

• Ask someone to lift up your thigh and bring your foot one step forward. Quickly, have them do the same thing with the other leg, then try to stand up.

• Bring your buttocks close to the edge of the chair. Keep your feet at least 8 inches apart, with one foot slightly in front of the other. Rock your trunk quickly back and forth a few times to build up momentum. On your last rock forward, bring your shoulders forward, just past your knees, and push down with your hands on the arms of the chair or the cushion while you straighten up to a standing position.

Mobility Devices

225. **Take a cane to help stabilize your walking when visiting unfamiliar places.** Usually, people will try to be more careful not to bump into you when they see a cane.

226. **If you use a cane, and you must go out in icy weather,** screw a removable ice gripper tip into the bottom of your cane or use a ski pole instead of a cane when walking on icy sidewalks.*

227. **If you use a cane in winter, and have difficulty gripping the cane handle while wearing mittens or gloves,** knit or crochet a small sleeve to fit snugly over the handle of the cane. The woolen glove and the woolen cover will work together to keep your hand from slipping.

228. **Clip a Super Light onto canes, walkers, and wheel-chairs for hands-free lighting.** Clip this high-intensity flashlight onto canes, walkers, and wheelchairs for convenient hands-free lighting. The light beam adjusts from flood to spotlight. It installs without tools. Two AAA batteries are included; a spare bulb sits inside the tail cap. The manufacturer provides a limited lifetime warranty.*

229. **Use a walking stick that resembles a shepherd's staff,** if you have trouble walking with a traditional cane but need support when you walk. The difference is that you hold the staff in front of you, and your elbow is bent at a 90-degree angle. The staff also helps you stand up straighter when your back muscles are weak. To see if walking with a staff helps you, get a broom or mop, cut the handle off, and put a rubber crutch protector on the end that touches the floor.

230. **Adapt a traditional walker for easier use:** Put 3-inch wheels on the front legs and tennis balls on the back legs of a walker, especially if you have thick or looped carpeting.

231. **Know when to let go.** Use it or lose it is a common motto but at some point, the effort involved to accomplish a task, such as walking, may far exceed any benefits of doing so. Don't think of using adaptive devices as giving in; think of it as expanding your ability to enjoy life. When an activity becomes difficult, seriously consider all your options. If you let go, you may find the assistance of devices such as walkers, wheelchairs, lifts, and scooters will help you conserve energy and actually make your life better and more enjoyable.*

232. **Consider using a wheeled walker.** Models are available with wheels and brakes, a seat in the middle for you to rest on, and a basket above the wheels where you can put loose items. You can hang a tote bag or a wicker bicycle basket from the top to keep important items handy, like your cordless telephone, a box of tissues, a pen, and a small notebook. To make it more secure, have a shoemaker make two special buckle straps for you to thread through the basket and attach to your walker (or to the handlebars of your three-wheeled scooter, if you use one).

233. **Three-wheeled scooters are narrower than most conventional wheelchairs, making them easier to get through doorways.** Some can be dismantled into three separate pieces for easy storage in the trunk of your car.

Outdoor Recreation

234. **For outdoor enjoyment, all-terrain and beach wheelchairs are available.** If you enjoy the outdoors often, consider purchasing your own. If you go on outdoor adventures only occasionally, consider rental equipment or look into accessibility options at federal, state, and local parks.*

235. **The Phil-E-Slide is an ergonomically designed patient lift system that may be helpful to caregivers and to people who are unable to move themselves.** The Phil-E-Slide system is made of ultra low-friction material that improves comfort and independence by enabling a person to transfer with significantly minimal effort.*

236. **Service dogs, similar to leader dogs for the blind, can help people with**

Parkinson's disease and other serious mobility problems. Service dogs can be trained to assist a person with balance, help her get out of a freeze, and assist if the person falls. The dogs have been shown to significantly reduce people's tendency to fall, and they provide a source of unconditional affection that can be greatly beneficial to anyone, regardless of impairment.*

Leisure and Recreational Activities

Reading

237. **Use a ruler or piece of paper as a guide to help your eyes track the lines on the page you are reading.**

238. **Use the eraser on a pencil or a rubber fingertip (like those used by secretaries and bookkeepers) to turn pages in a book.**

239. **Purchase a full-page sheet magnifier** made of wafer-thin plastic that magnifies an entire page at one time. Or, use a hand-held magnifier to help you look up telephone numbers, scan maps, examine

floor plans, read operating instructions or stock market reports, handle hobby and needlecraft projects, and make other tasks easier. Lighted magnifiers may be found at book, craft, or home health stores.

240. **Check out the large-print book selection at your local library.** Take advantage of the library's collection of large-print and audio books. The *Large-Type Books in Print* directory includes books and periodicals published in large print. This reference book is available at most major libraries.

241. **The Book Clubs division of Double-day & Company has a large-print home library.** A wide range of full-length hardcover best-sellers, including fiction, mystery, romance, and how-to titles, are offered.*

242. **Talking Newspapers for people with physical or visual disabilities.** The National Federation of the Blind has created the Newsline for the Blind, a free service accessible by any touch-tone telephone 24 hours a day. People who are blind, disabled, or unable to read

the newspaper on their own can call a toll-free access line and listen to articles from daily and Sunday issues of a local, regional, or national newspaper such as the *Chicago Tribune,* the *Los Angeles Times,* the *Washington Post, USA Today,* the *New York Times,* and the *Wall Street Journal.* Touch-tone menus allow users to jump from one section of the paper to another, from one article to another, or from one newspaper to another. Personal adjustments can be made to reading speed and voice, or paused to hear the pronunciation or spelling of any given word. To access the service, you must have a physical or visual disability that prevents you from reading a newspaper. To obtain an application, contact the National Federation of the Blind. You will be issued an identification number and a security code, which you must enter each time you use the service.*

243. **Enroll in the Talking Book Program.** If you have a documented physical or visual disability, you may qualify for the Talking Book Program of the National Library Service for the Blind and Physically Handicapped (NLS). Choose from more than 159,000 biographies, best

sellers, classics, poetry, mysteries, how-to, and other books, as well as 70 popular magazines. The special tape recorder needed to play the tapes as well as accessories like headphones, remote control units, and amplifiers are available from the Talking Books program. All items and services connected with this program are free. Even the postage on the books is paid. You are eligible for Talking Books if you meet any of the following criteria:

• You are unable to read standard print without aids or devices other than glasses or contact lenses.

• You have a visual acuity of less than 20/200 or a visual field of 20 degrees or less with correction.

• You are unable to hold a book or turn a page.

• You have a temporary loss of vision or use of your hands.

• You have a medically documented reading disability.*

244. **If you listen to audio books, position the tape recorder and stand/table in a convenient position that you can reach.** Then, mark the location of the stand on the floor with masking tape so that anyone can easily set up the audio books for you.

245. **Find out if your local radio stations broadcast book readings.** Public radio stations often have a program when a chapter is read from a current novel each day.

246. **The Internet now offers books in electronic versions** including MP3 formats that can be easily downloaded and played back at your convenience.

247. **Make reading while lying flat in bed easier with Bed Specs or Prism glasses.** You wear them just like a regular pair of glasses (they may even be worn over your existing glasses), and they allow you to see a book or television screen even when you are lying on your back. The glasses may be adjusted to any head width.*

248. **L-Bow 4-in-1 Blanket is the perfect for someone who sits in a wheelchair or spends time in bed.** This soft, cuddly 60 by 72-inch fleece blanket can be used as a throw, or you can slip your arms through the built-in sleeves and tuck the blanket around your shoulders for warmth while leaving your arms and hands are free to knit, read, do crossword puzzles, and other sedentary activities. A foot pouch at the bottom of the blanket is a handy foot warmer. When not in use, the 4-In-1 Blanket folds into a plush pillow that can sit on your couch, chair, or bed. The 4-In-1 Blanket is machine washable, comes in red, navy, and hunter green.*

Watching Television

249. **Purchase or make a holder for eye-glasses, flashlight, pencil, crossword puzzle book, and other items.** For your bed, create pockets on one end of a length of material about twice the length of the distance between mattress and floor. Place half of the material, the end without the pockets, between the mattress and the box spring allowing

the pockets to hang down the side of the bed to hold your things.

For the armrest of your favorite chair, create your own saddlebag-style holder for TV and VCR remote control devices. To make a holder, select two hand towels that fit with your decor and room colors and sew them together at one end to make one long piece. Then, fold up each end to create pockets to hold your remotes. If possible, divide one of the pockets in half and use it to hold a pencil and note pad. You may also want to secure your holder to the arm of your couch or chair with a few stitches or Velcro. You may find a commercial version of these holders in specialty catalogs, on the Internet, or in discount department stores.

250. **Purchase a universal remote control and program it to operate both the VCR and the TV.** Universal remotes cost less than $20 and can be used in the home and elsewhere to operate the TV, VCR, stereo, and DVD player.

251. **Use a large-button adapter for your remote control,** if you have trouble with fine motor movements. Some fit over and snap onto the small remote buttons or your regular remote; others

are universal and replace your standard remote control.*

252. **Take a plain adhesive-backed label and write the cable channels and their numbers on it.** Put the label on the back of your remote control, where you can easily consult it. Now, you won't have to remember all the channel numbers or page through a *TV Guide* or newspaper listing whenever you want to watch a program.

253. **Calming videos and DVDs provide respite.** Videos and DVDs with nature themes can provide natural relaxation and entertainment for people with dementia and give their care partner a little break. Sit down and take a soothing trip through a garden, visit a country pond, watch an aquarium, or just enjoy the warm coziness of a country hearth. *Note:* Videos and DVDs are no substitute for care or supervision.*

To have a constant supply of new videos and DVDs without running to and from the store, consider signing up for a subscription service that offers unlimited rentals that you can keep as long as you want. Blockbuster, Wal-Mart, and Netflix (www.netflix.com) all have rental plans. Monthly rates run $15.50 to $30.

254. **Family videos and DVDs provide comfort to one with memory loss.** Family videos and DVDS featuring familiar voices and faces are a source of comfort to one with memory loss. If a loved one is lost in the past, transfer old photos or movies of a time they remember to video or DVD.

Playing Games

255. **Try doing crossword puzzles or playing games like Scrabble, Scattergories, and Taboo** to help exercise your ability to remember words. Playing Trivial Pursuit is another great way to keep your memory in shape. Deluxe and adaptive games are available for people with low vision, poor hand coordination, and other disabilities.*

256. **If you enjoy watching game shows on television, play along at home.** Say the answers aloud while watching *Wheel of Fortune, Jeopardy!,* or *Who Wants to Be a Millionaire.*

257. **Use jumbo playing cards,** which are easier to use than regular cards; they are available at most drug stores or toy stores. Some "crooked decks" are available that make it easier to grasp individual cards, and automatic card shufflers can aid with that task.*

258. **To make holding cards easier,** purchase a card holder. Or, take an old shoebox, remove the top, and put the bottom of the box inside the cover. The space between the cover and the side of the shoebox holds the cards nicely.*

Improving Memory and Concentration

259. **Write yourself reminder notes and put them where you'll see them.** For example, if you have an appointment in the morning, tape a reminder note to the bathroom mirror so that you will see it first thing.

260. **Set an alarm on your computer, microwave, watch, or pager to remind you to take medications, to drink or eat something, or to exercise.** Leave a note on the alarm or the

computer, so that you know what to do when you turn off the alarm.

261. **To help with time and sequencing, create a calendar for the month with large squares for each day.** Write down appointments, special events, and symbols for the weather in the appropriate square.

262. **To keep track of daily events, purchase a spiral notebook.** Start a new page for each day. Begin the day by recording the time of day and what happened. For example: "8:00 Breakfast (French Toast); 9:00 Talked to sister Ann."

263. **Keep your memory active by reviewing the day's news events with a friend or neighbor.** Read the daily newspaper together and then quiz each other on details of the stories that most interest you.

264. **To help you remember whether or not you have locked the door say out loud, "I'm locking the door" as you lock up.**

265. **We often think of things that we need to remember at inopportune times,** like in a darkened movie theater or out walking the dog. If it's inconvenient to write yourself a note, take off your watch or wedding band and put it on the opposite hand or double-knot your shoelaces. That way, you will give yourself a reminder that there is something you want to remember, and you can make a note of it at a more convenient time.

RESOURCES

4-In-1 Fleece Blanket

L-Bow Mittens
888-648-8367
www.lbow.com

Assistance Dogs

Assistance Dog United Campaign
1221 Sebastopol Road
Santa Rosa, CA95407
800284-DOGS (3647)
www.assistancedogunitedcampaign.org

Canine Companions for Independence
National Headquarters & Northwest Regional
 Center
2965 Dutton Avenue
P.O. Box 446
Santa Rosa, CA95402-0446
Phone 707-577-1700
TTY 707-577-1756
www.caninecompanions.org

Paws with a Cause
4646 South Division
Wayland, MI49348
800-253-7297
www.pawswithacause.com

Automatic Card Shuffler

Easy Street Co.
509 Birchwood Court
Raymore, MO64083
800-959-EASY; (3279)
www.easystreetco.com

Bed Specs or Prism Glasses

Allegro Medical
800-861-3211
www.allegromedical.com

Big-button Remote Control

Dynamic Living
428 Hayden Station Road
Windsor, CT06095-1302
888-940-0605
www.dynamic-living.com

Independent Living Aids, Inc.
200 Robbins Lane
Jericho, NY11753-2341
800-537-2118
516-752-3135
www.independentliving.com

Sammons Preston Rolyan
An AbilityOne Company
270 Remington Boulevard, Suite C
Bolingbrook, IL60440-3593
Worldwide Telephone: 630-226-1300
TDD 800-325-1745
www.sammonspreston.com

Calming Videos and DVDs

Ageless Design, Inc.
12633159th Court
North Jupiter, FL33478-6669
800-752-3238
561-745-0210

www.alzstore.com

Crooked Playing Cards

Uncle's Games
3808 North Sullivan Road,
Building 8
Spokane Valley, WA99216
866-826-6959
www.unclesgames.com

Deluxe and Adaptive Games

Independent Living Aids, Inc.
200 Robbins Lane
Jericho, NY11753
800-537-2118
www.IndependentLiving.com

Large Print Books

Doubleday Large Print
Doubleday Direct, Inc.
Member Services
1225 South Market Street
Mechanicsburg, PA17055
www.doubledaylargeprint.com

Mobility Equipment, Adaptive Devices and Independent Living Aids

Amigo Mobility International, Inc.
6693 Dixie Highway
Bridgeport, MI48722-9725
800-MY-AMIGO (692-6446)
www.myamigo.com

Sammons Preston Rolyan
An AbilityOne Company
270 Remington Boulevard, Suite C
Bolingbrook, IL60440-3593
Worldwide Telephone: 630-226-1300
TDD 800-325-1745
www.sammonspreston.com

Spinlife.com
1108 City Park Avenue
Columbus, OH43206
800-850-0335
614-449-8123
www.spinlife.com

Outdoor Accessibility Options

Access to Recreation, Inc.
8 Sandra Court

Newbury Park, CA91320
800-634-4351
www.accesstr.com

Deming Designs Inc.
1090 Cobblestone Drive
Pensacola, FL32514
850-478-5765
www.beachwheelchair.com

Natural Access
P.O. Box 5729
Santa Monica, CA90409-5729
800-411-7789
310-392-9864
www.natural-access.com

Phil-E-Slide

Phil-E-Slide, USA
389 Main Street
Salem, NH03079
866-675-4338
603-328-9213
www.phil-e-slide-us.com

Playing Card Holder

Maddak, Inc.
661 Route 23 South

Wayne, NJ07470
973-628-7600
www.ableware.com

Always Something Brilliant
8141 N. I-70 Frontage Road
Arvada, CO80002
www.alwaysbrilliant.com

Spiky Plus Traction Grips

Thomas Fetterman, Inc.
1680 Hillside Road
Southampton, PA18966
888-582-5544
www.fetterman-crutches.com

Super Light

Access with Ease, Inc.
P.O. Box 1150
Chino Valley, AZ86323
800-531-9479; 602-636-9469
www.store.yahoo.com/capability

Talking Book Program

The National Library Service for the Blind and
 Physically Handicapped
Library of Congress

Washington, DC20542
800-424-9100
www.loc.gov/nls

Talking Newspapers

National Federation of the Blind
1800 Johnson Street
Baltimore, MD21230
410-659-9314
www.nfb.org

CHAPTER 7

Handling Medical Issues

Few of us are prepared for the diagnosis of a serious chronic illness like Parkinson's disease. However, as the reality of the diagnosis begins to take hold, you quickly learn that healthcare providers and medical professionals will now be a part of your life. Dealing with doctors, pharmacists, and therapists—not to mention all the new medical terminology, procedures, and tests—can be a real challenge. Keeping organized and taking an active role in managing your healthcare will give you back some control over your illness and assure family members that you are coping well with your new reality.

Managing your medical care will be easier if all your doctors and specialists belong to the same medical practice or HMO, because all your medical records will be in one place. In addition, seeing other specialists in the group (orthopedists,physiatrists,occupational/physical therapists, speech/language pathologists, and psychologists/psychiatrists) can reduce the hassles of obtaining referrals and filling out endless paperwork at new doctors' offices. Find out, too, if your insurance covers home health services for medical management in the home, physical therapy visits, and so on. You may be surprised at what is covered.

A healthcare provider's bedside manner can be extremely important. Choose a doctor you like and with whom you have a good rapport. Research shows that patients who are satisfied with their physicians are healthier overall than those who are not. If a friend or acquaintance recommends a doctor, keep in mind that you may have a different experience, opinion, or preference. If your doctor doesn't treat you with respect, listen to you, or see you as a whole person—as an individual, a family member, a person with a career and a social life—find one who does. Obtain a copy of the Patient's Bill of Rights and make sure that your healthcare providers adhere to it. Learning to stick up for yourself and be your own advocate can give you back some of the power and control that PD takes away.

Another way to get involved in your own healthcare is to learn more than you ever wanted to know about PD. The American Parkinson's Disease Association (APDA) and the National Parkinson Foundation (NPF) are wonderful resources for accurate, up-to-date information. Enlist your friends and family members to do research, too. It will give you all something positive to do. Collect information from newspapers, magazines, and medical journals. If there is a university near your home, visit the medical-school library or search for reputable resources on the Internet. Share information and learn together. Bring articles and information to your next doctor's appointment, so that you can discuss the findings and see how they relate to your case. You may even find that you've read medical journal articles before your doctor has had a chance to read them. It never hurts to be proactive when it comes to your health. Be sure that you and your family know how any prescribed medications work, what the side effects are, and which side effects you should report to your doctor. Do not take any medication, including nonprescription products such as vitamins, dietary supplements, allergy and cold medicines, pain relievers, or herbal remedies, without first consulting your doctor.

This chapter contains many more tips and ideas to help you manage your medical care.

Record Keeping and Research

266. **Compile your own personal medical file.** Purchase a three-ring binder and several sheets with divider tabs.

Use a three-hole punch so that you can insert any kind of paper into the notebook. Organize the binder into sections:

- Family health history.

- Past illnesses.

- Dated summaries of office appointments, tests, treatments, surgical procedures, and hospitalizations, including copies of test results.

- Prescription log, with details about the names and dosages of all your medications, including nonprescription medications and vitamin supplements, and notes on why, when, and how often you take the drugs.

- Symptom log, to track how you feel before and after the introduction of a new medication, as well as recording any new symptoms or side effects.

Keeping a symptom log is important because, if you don't write them down, you may report only those symptoms to the doctor that you actually feel while you're in the office for an appointment.

• Question and answer log, to keep track of questions you have for your doctor, along with the answers you receive.

As the years pass, this file will be an invaluable reference. Keep it up to date and thorough. Bring it with you to all medical appointments, especially to your first appointment with a new doctor. The file doesn't take the place of your original medical records, but it will help doctors get a quick overview and more thorough understanding of your history of treatment.

267. **You may want to purchase "Your Personal Health and Medical History," published by Planet Media Group and HealthHistory.com. The organizer is designed for people with long-term medical needs and is divided into ten categories (such as personal information, medications, hospitalizations, emergency contacts, etc.). The organizer also contains detailed forms that are easy to fill out and 18 legal documents (including**

Power of Attorney, healthcare directives, etc.). You can purchase the organizer in a three-ringed binder, a bound work-book, or on CD. The cost is between $12 and $50.*

268. **Get copies of all your official medical records** and keep them in a special section of your personal medical file. More than half the states have enacted laws giving patients access to their hos-pital and physician records. You may have more difficulty in states that haven't enacted such laws, but no state specifically denies access to your records. There will likely be a cost to obtain your medical records, which varies from state to state. Keep all medical documents in a central location where they can be found easily, and let family members and helpers know where the file is in case it is needed in an emergency.

269. **Carry an index card in your purse or wallet with a list of your medications** (including dosages), and any allergies or special medical conditions you have. You will be asked for this information over and over again, and having it on

paper is better than relying on memory. Use a second card for the names and phone numbers of your primary care physician, your specialists, nurses, medical supply company, clergy, emergency contacts, and the like. Carry both cards at all times. Also, consider keeping this information in a small electronic planner or hand-held personal data assistant like a Palm Pilot. Give a duplicate set of these cards to your helpers, family members, or close friends.

270.   **Computer users can use the Internet to access the world's largest medical library—the National Library of Medicine** in Bethesda, Maryland. At this site, you will find health, treatment, and medication information in easy-to-understand layman's terms. For more information, contact the Office of Public Information at the National Institutes of Health.*

For information about PD-related tests, procedures, or treatments, call your local Parkinson's support group. With a little education, you can learn to phrase your questions in medical terms that doctors understand. You also can learn more about what symptoms you should report to your doctor.

Doctors' Appointments

271. **Mornings and right after the lunch hour are often the best times for scheduling a doctor's appointment.** At those times, appointments are more likely to be running closer to schedule. Also, consider the time of day when you are most energetic or when your medication leaves you at your peak.

272. **If you are anxious to see the doctor soon,** tell the receptionist. Ask if there is an early opening due to a cancellation; if not, ask to be notified if someone does cancel. Ask to be put on the "short list." Call back in a few days, if you have not heard from the receptionist.

273. **If you have a lot to talk about with your doctor, make a consultation appointment** so that the doctor will allow enough time to meet with you without being hurried. Give the receptionist the option of lengthening your appointment or scheduling a second appoint-

ment slot for you. You should be willing to pay for this extra time.

274.   **Be clear about what you want to say to the doctor,** and try not to introduce extraneous information into your description of symptoms or other concerns. Write down your points in advance. It can be helpful to prepare a brief but accurate progress report, answering such questions as: How closely have you been following your treatment plan? How have you been feeling? How many hours a day do you feel "on" and "off?" Have you had any specific problems? What has been happening in your life? It may be helpful to have a family member or helper contribute to your progress report, recording their perceptions of your "on" and "off" times. Having more than one perspective often can give the physician a clearer picture. Remember, your doctor sees you only for a short amount of time; to adequately manage your PD, he needs to know how things have gone at home since your last appointment.

275.   **Pay careful attention to your sleep patterns.** If you tend to fall asleep

during a particular activity, tell your doctor. You might be experiencing sleep attacks, which are different from normal sleepiness. Also, keep track of any hallucinations or delusions you might be experiencing. Medications can sometimes cause nocturnal wanderings, hallucinations, delusions, or other problems. Adjusting your dosage of a particular medication or adding a new prescription might help with those symptoms. If your sleep is still disturbed even after following your doctor's recommendations about the timing of your medication doses, consider getting an examination by a sleep specialist trained in managing patients with neurologic disorders.

276. **Bring pen and paper, and write down what your doctor says.** Remembering everything your doctor advises can be a challenge. Sometimes it can be helpful to bring someone with you to the doctor's appointment to serve as a second set of ears. However, that strategy won't work if you feel unable to speak as freely to your doctor when a friend or family member is present. If you do bring someone along, be sure

to communicate openly and honestly with your doctor.

277. **Ask for clarification,** if for any reason you are not satisfied with the explanations your doctor gives you. If your doctor uses medical terms that you do not understand, or if you are not sure how serious your diagnosis is, say so. Say, for example, "Could you say that in layman's terms?" or "I'm not sure I understood that. Would you explain it again?" If you wish to hear another opinion, ask for a second opinion from another physician. Don't worry about hurting your doctor's feelings; any reasonable practitioner should understand your desire to cover all the bases. Trust your instincts.

278. **If you have a medical test, protect yourself and your family by asking questions.** Are the tests processed in the office or are they sent out to an off-site lab? How long will it take to get the results back? When can you expect a call? Can you get a copy of the test results to keep in your home medical file? If you don't hear from the doctor in the specified time, call until you get the in-

formation you need. Don't assume that "no news is good news." Sometimes, test orders can be misplaced or delayed, so even if the doctor's office says they will contact you with the results, take the initiative to find out.

279. **If your doctor recommends a particular treatment, ask to be put in touch with other PD patients who have undergone the same treatment** or discuss it in a PD support group with others. Find out how effective it was and whether they had any adverse reactions to it.

Medications

280. **Always ask your doctor or pharmacist for published information (a brochure from the manufacturer, for example) on any drug you've been prescribed.** If you have trouble reading printed material, such as a prescription medication insert, enlarge it. Photocopy machines at copy shops, libraries and post offices are capable of enlarging print to make it easier to read, or scan it into the computer or use a magnifying glass to help you read.

281. **Ask specifically about every drug's side effects,** the amount of time it will take for the drug to reach full effectiveness in your body, and whether any potentially harmful interactions can occur between the drugs you are taking (both prescription and nonprescription). Ask if you can try a 1-week supply of the drug to see how well you tolerate it before purchasing an entire month's supply.

282. **Consult the Physician's Desk Reference (PDR),** available on-line, for specific information about your medications.*

283. **Start a new medication as early in the day as possible.** If you have an adverse reaction, it will be easier to reach the doctor.

284. **Ask your doctor or pharmacist to write the number of times a day you should take your medication.** It is easy to misinterpret dosing instructions when they are written as hourly intervals (e.g., one tablet every 6 hours). But few people misinterpret instructions that specify daily frequency

(e.g., one tablet four times per day). Write out the dosage schedule and carry it with you. Check off each dose as you take it. If a particular drug must be taken in the middle of the night, ask if an alternative prescription is available that is more convenient to take.

285. **A "talking" pill bottle verbally instructs you about your medication.** Have your pharmacist record the name of the medication, the dosage, and the frequency which you should take your medication into the cap. (You or a family member or friend can also do this.) Whenever you need a reminder, just push the button and the instructions will be repeated for you.*

286. **Familiarize yourself with some of the abbreviations used on prescriptions:**

- QD=every day

- BID=two times per day

- TID=three times per day

- QID=four times per day

- PO=by mouth

- AC=before meals

- PC=after meals

- HS=at bedtime

287. **Choose one pharmacy to fill all your prescriptions.** If you are receiving drugs from more than one doctor, no one physician will have a complete list of your medications. Avoid scattering your prescriptions among several pharmacies. Instead, pick one that fits your needs and stick to it. That way, there will be a complete record of your prescriptions and drug allergies on file in one place, and your pharmacist can easily check that a new prescription does not adversely interact with a medication you are already taking. Also, find out if your pharmacy has a computer system that will automatically generate alerts when any of your prescriptions have harmful interactions.

288. **Ask your pharmacist for non-childproof bottles with easy-open caps;** this will make it easier if you have trouble opening traditional prescription bottles. Some pharmacies also offer large-print labels that are much easier to read.

289. **Save time and energy by having your prescriptions mailed from the pharmacy to your home.**

290. **Keep a list of your daily medications taped to the refrigerator, microwave, or medicine cabinet.** List the time of day, name of the drug, and dose. Check off each dose as you take it.

291. **Use a weekly pill organizer with morning, noon, evening, and bedtime slots for each day.** At the beginning of each week, fill the organizer with your medications. You can also use a clean egg carton to organize your pills.*

292. **Keep track of medication times by using one of the following methods:**

• **Purchase a digital sports watch with a countdown repeat timer;** this works well if you need to take medication at a regular interval, such as every 4 hours. With this feature, the watch beeps after 4 hours, then automatically starts counting down to the next 4-hour interval. They come in both men's and women's styles, with metal or nylon bands. If you don't want to be disturbed by the watch beeping in the middle of the night, take it off and leave it in another room.

• **Purchase a "double-alarm" alarm clock.** Because morning pills and evening pills are the easiest to remember, set the alarm to go off, for example, at 12:00P.M. and 4:00P.M. After the alarm rings at 4:00P.M., press the reset button and the alarm will automatically sound the next day at 12:00P.M.

• **Program your cell-phone alarm.** Most cell phones allow you to set several alarms for daily or intermittent reminders; they also may have a quick alarm that will ring in a set period of time (such as every 4 hours). Use one or a combination of these alarms to remind you of your medication schedule.

• **An electronic timer reminds you when to take your medication.** The MedGlider System has three alarm types (beeping alarm, voice alarm, or visual alarm) that can each be programmed to alert you up to three times at 1-minute intervals and for four dose settings. The LCD screen is large, clear, and easy to read, displaying the current time, the number of daily doses selected, a missed pill alert, and an alarm mode. It has large buttons and separate hour and minute buttons for easy programming. The MedGlider timer, which requires two AAA batteries (not included), may be attached to a four-compartment pillbox and is small enough to conceal in a coat pocket or purse.*

• **A vibrating locket discreetly reminds you to take medication.** The Chronostone Personal Timer is a convenient and attractive alternative for aiding women in taking medication on time. Set the alarm, and the locket silently vibrates at the same time each day, with a "second chance alarm."*

293. **Take a hard-to-swallow pill with a spoonful of apple-sauce or pudding.** For more tips on making swallowing pills easier, see the section on swallowing in

the Managing Mealtime Madness chapter.

294. **Be sure to discuss the specifics of pill splitting with your doctor.** Sometimes, your doctor might prescribe a dosage that is smaller than what is commercially available and instruct you to split pills in half. Or, to save you money, your doctor might prescribe a higher dosage than you need and recommend that you split the pills. You might be tempted to split pills if they are too large to swallow easily—*do not* split or crush up hard-to-swallow pills without first checking with your physician. Some pills are enteric coated (to bypass your stomach and be absorbed by your intestines) or time released and should never be split. If you split pills, up to 20 percent of the pill's mass may be lost as dust and fragments (even if you use a pill-splitter); be sure to ask your doctor if the effectiveness of your medicine would be diminished by splitting. If you do split pills, split them one at a time, as you need them; the rough edges of split pills will erode and lose even more of the

medication if they are put back in the bottle.

295. **Never use household silverware to administer medication.** You could be receiving an incorrect dosage. Always use an oral dropper, cylindrical dosing spoon, syringe, or plastic medicine cup. You can find these devices at a pharmacy or discount department store.

296. **Talk to your doctor if you are troubled by a dry mouth.** Many medications and medical conditions can cause dry mouth syndrome. Normal amounts of saliva are important to maintain healthy teeth and gums; a lack of saliva increases the incidence of decay and periodontal disease (gum disease). Saliva also aids in swallowing, digestion, and the ability to speak normally. Because dry mouth is very common, products have been developed for the treatment of this condition; many are sold over the counter in drugstores. Consult your doctor or dentist to discuss this common condition and possible treatments appropriate for you. In the meantime, keep a

glass of water nearby; sip from it regularly during the day, swishing the water around in your mouth to moisten your gums.

297. **Tell your doctor if you experience dramatic changes in your mood** during the day or from day to day. As many as 50 percent of people with PD have mood swings. Mood swings can be caused by the disease itself or by medications. Your doctor might alter your medications or recommend that you exercise regularly, start a new project, get involved in a support group, or talk with a therapist.

298. **Keep track of how you feel after eating various kinds of meals, and discuss any dietary restrictions you should observe while on your medications with your doctor.** The effectiveness of some PD medications is affected by diet; for example, the absorption of levodopa is delayed if it is taken with a meal rich in protein. On the other hand, many people do not tolerate levodopa on an empty stomach; they experience nausea and vomiting. If taking medications causes nausea, try taking

it with ginger ale or a gingersnap cookie.

299. **If you are taking Sinemet try dissolving it in a sugared, carbonated beverage** like Sprite, Coca-Cola, or ginger ale to optimize its effectiveness.

300. **If you are staying in the hospital, ask your doctor to write an order for you to be able to take your own Parkinson's disease medications.** This is important, because sometimes it's difficult to get medication administered exactly on time while you are in the hospital. Generally, if medication is scheduled to be given at 1:00P.M., it can be administered between 12:00 noon and 2:00P.M. and still be considered on time. For people with PD, 10 to 15 minutes can be the difference between staying "on" and going "off." If you're admitted to a general medical unit, ask to speak with the head nurse about the importance of timing your PD medications to control your symptoms. Give the doctors and nurses a copy of your normal medication regime. Make sure a note is recorded in your chart so that you can give yourself your medications when you need them.

301. **If the person with PD begins hallucinating,** try to explain that the medicine isn't working and is causing the hallucination. Keep notes on what time of day the hallucinations occur; also record what was taken and when the medications were last taken. This will help the doctor if the medications need to be adjusted. Adjusting the medications may not make the hallucinations disappear, but they may be less disturbing. (For example, if the person sees large green giants, medication adjustment may cause the person to see little green ants.)**

Managing Your Home Healthcare

302. **Buy a digital thermometer, not a glass one.** Digital thermometers are easier to read and are safer than glass because they won't break in your mouth.

303. **Use a microwaveable heat pad for backaches;** they are safer to use than electric heating pads. They cool down gradually, like a hot water bottle, and won't burn the skin.

304. **Wrap a Chux pad around a warm compress;** the compress will stay warmer and the moisture won't seep out onto garments or furniture. You can purchase Chux (a plastic-backed pad with an absorbent cotton lining typically used in bed for incontinence) or similar pads at drug stores.

305. **To make a cold compress,** wet a washcloth and keep it in a storage bag in your freezer. When you need a compress, remove it from the freezer and allow it to thaw slightly. Then, place it where you need it. When you have finished, return the damp wash-cloth to the freezer; it will be ready to use again the next time you need it.

306. **Use an inflatable neck cushion** to rest your head while lying in bed or sitting in your armchair. A U-shaped or dog bone-shaped pillow may also provide you with comfortable neck support.

307. **Use pillows to position the person with PD on his side in bed;** thera-pists can show you how. Instead of

buying big pillows, roll up towels and hold the roll in place with rubber bands; these towel pillows can be laundered easily, unlike large pillows.**

308. **Create a makeshift backrest** for the person who must stay in bed and would like to sit up. First, remove the pillows from the bed. Then, take a straight-backed chair and turn it upside down and place it on the mattress where the pillows were. The front edge of the seat will touch the mattress, the legs of the chair will be pointing in the air toward the headboard or wall, and the top portion of the back of the chair will rest on the mattress, creating a slanted surface to cushion with pillows and lean on.**

309. **If you have leg cramps,** a quick way to relieve them is to bite your lower lip while pinching your upper lip. It may look silly but it helps some people.

310. **If your arms feel cold,** pull a pair of children's leg warmers up your arm all the way to the underarm and

shoulder. If your legs are cold, purchase a pair of adult-size leg warmers
for your legs and knees. If your feet
are cold in bed, wear regular short
sport socks; if the elastic around the
ankle is too tight, clip it to relieve any
constriction.

311. **If you use a wheelchair or a
scooter,** try out different wheelchair
cushions until you find the one that
is most comfortable for you. Consult
your physical therapist for recommendations, and spend some time in your
hospital's home health or rehab store
trying out different cushions. You
spend a lot of time in your chair, so
make sure you are comfortable.

312. **To relieve constipation:**

• Drink at least eight 8-ounce glasses of
water every day

• Add one cup of unprocessed bran cere-
al to your daily diet or add bran powder
to non-bran cereals, applesauce, or soup.

• Sit comfortably on a low commode with knees drawn up to help the abdominal muscles pass the stool.

• Discuss other possible remedies with your doctor; this is important because the frequent use of laxatives, suppositories, and enemas can cause additional health problems.

313. **If you are concerned about your safety** or the safety of someone else around the house, you may want to consider a service like Lifeline, a 24-hour emergency response system service provided by many community hospitals. This service utilizes a communicator unit that is hooked up to your phone, plus a portable emergency help call button that you wear at all times. When you push the button, two-way communication between you and the Response Center is immediately activated through a powerful speakerphone in the communicator unit. When you subscribe to Lifeline service, you provide a list of people to be contacted in case of an emergency. When you activate the help button, the staff at the Response Center asks the nature of the problem, whom you wish

them to contact, or if you need emergency medical assistance. Health-Watch offers similar services. Check with your local hospital to find out if one of these programs or something similar is available in your area.*

314. **Alert rescue workers to illnesses and/or allergies in an emergency situation.** MedicAlert, a nonprofit membership-based organization, provides individual subscribers with small, wearable ID tags marked with the users' medical conditions and personal identification numbers. These football-shaped ID tags or "emblems" are a little more than an inch long and can be worn in a variety of styles, including bracelets, necklaces, or a sport band. In the event of an emergency, paramedics familiar with the Medic Alert emblem can contact the 24-hour Emergency Response Center's toll-free number, give the user's name, and receive pertinent health information. MedicAlert will then transfer the user's medical records to the hospital emergency department and also notify the user's family. The basic membership is $35 for the first year and $20 for

subsequent years, with your choice of emblem included.*

If you should wear a medical alert/identification tag but refrain because you don't like how they look, a number of fine jewelry styles for both men and women are available. Bracelets, pendants, chains, and medallions are made of sterling silver, gold, and platinum; some may be enhanced with precious stones.*

315.   **Assistance for paying for the high cost of drugs.** Services are available to help people of any age, people with disabilities, and people with low incomes locate the Patient Assistance Programs offered by many pharmaceutical companies. These programs provide free or reduced-cost medication to people who qualify. The Medicine Program is a volunteer organization that works in cooperation with the physician to assist patients who may qualify to enroll in one or more of the many Patient Assistance Programs available nationwide.*

316.   **To purchase home medical supplies,** check the Yellow Pages in your phone

book for listings under First Aid Supplies, Medical Supplies, Surgical Appliances, and Physicians and Surgeons—Equipment & Supplies. Usually, the kinds of outlets that offer home medical supplies are pharmacies, home healthcare stores (often affiliated with local hospitals), and surgical supply stores. You may also find many items in medical supply catalogs or online stores.*

317. **If you need special medical equipment for only a short time,** look into borrowing the equipment from local sources. Contact agencies like the Red Cross, Salvation Army, Visiting Nurse Service, home health agencies, churches, senior centers, and your local APDA chapter.

RESOURCES

Health History

Planet Media Group
13515 Old Dock Road
Orlando, FL32828
888-669-9697
www.HealthHistory.com

Health Reference Web Sites

National Institutes of Health
www.medlineplus.gov

Physician's Desk Reference
www.pdrhealth.com/drug_info

U.S. National Library of Medicine
www.nlm.nih.gov

MedGlider System

Dynamic Living
428 Hayden Station Road
Windsor, CT06095-1302
888-940-0605
www.dynamic-living.com

Medical Alert Systems

Health Watch Inc.
6400 Park of Commerce Boulevard, Suite 1-A
Boca Raton, FL33487
800-226-8100
www.health-watch.com

Lifeline
800-380-3111
www.lifelinesys.com

Medic Alert
2005 Sheppard Avenue East,
Suite 800
Toronto, ONM2J 5B4
Canada
888-633-4298
www.medicalert.com

Medical ID Jewelry

Medic ID International
P.O. Box 571687
Tarzana, CA91357
818-705-0595
800-926-3342
www.medicid.com

Medical Supplies

Allegro Medical
1733 East McKellips,
Suite 110
Tempe, AZ85281
800-861-3211
www.allegromedical.com

RehabMart.com: Discount Rehab Superstore
150 Sagewood Drive
Winterville, GA30683-1563
800-827-8283

706-283-3242
www.rehabmart.com

Sammons Preston Rolyan
An AbilityOne Company
270 Remington Boulevard,
Suite C Bolingbrook, IL60440-3593
Worldwide Telephone: 630-226-1300
TDD 800-325-1745
www.sammonspreston.com

Medication Reminder Tools

Easy Street Co.
509 Birchwood Court
Raymore, MO64083
800-959-EASY (3279)
www.easystreetco.com

Improvements Catalog
800-642-2112
www.improvementscatalog.com

The Medicine Program

The Medicine Program
P.O. Box 1089
Poplar Bluff, MO63902-1089
Toll-free: 866-694-3893
www.themedicineprogram.com

Talking Pill Bottle

Easy Street Co.
509 Birchwood Court
Raymore, MO64083
800-959-EASY (3279)
www.easystreetco.com

Vibrating Locket

Easy Street Co
509 Birchwood Court
Raymore, MO64083
800-959-EASY (3279)
www.easystreetco.com

CHAPTER 8

Getting Out and About

Don't let Parkinson's disease (PD) limit your world. With a little forethought, you will find that you can get out and do more than you might think. Before you leave the house, take a few minutes to think over the errands you have to run. Ask yourself, "Is it a good time of day to be going to the library or post office?" or "Will the drive-up windows at the bank be open?" Rearrange the order of your stops to make errands most convenient for you. If you're prone to forget the sequence, write it down. Leave low-priority stops at the bottom of the list, so that if you get tired, you can leave them for another time.

Parkinson's disease and some of the medications used to control it can have an impact on your perception and reaction time and possibly affect your ability to drive safely. Be realistic about your abilities; have someone else drive you if necessary. Discuss with a doctor any concerns you might have about driving, and see if adjusting your medications can improve your ability to drive.

With a little extra planning, a realistic itinerary, and some creativity, you can still get out and do many of the things you want to.

Errands and Outings

318. **Plan ahead before going out.** Put your credit card in an easily accessible place, get out the money you will need for using public transportation, and begin to make out a check if you feel it takes too much time to do in the checkout lane. (If you fill in the receiver's name and date, then all you have to do is sign the check and ask the cashier to fill in the amount. When you get home, use the store receipt to fill in the amount of the check in the ledger.

319. **Before going out, call ahead to the restaurant, theater, gallery, and other places, and ask if the establishment is accessible (including the restrooms);** ask about parking facilities, about which is the most convenient entrance, and so on. When you reach your destination, keep seating arrangements in mind. If you

use a wheelchair, ask for a table instead of a booth. If you are going to a theater, but have trouble moving to accommodate others trying to reach seats further into your row, try to sit in a front row, or reserve the end seat and wait until the entire row has been seated before you sit down.

320. **Use a walkie-talkie set so that you are never out of touch** when you go shopping with friends or relatives in large stores and malls. Otherwise, it can be easy to lose track of each other. Some cell phone services now offer this feature.

321. **If your destination lacks convenient seating—such as a museum, park, shopping mall, or other public place—bring your own.** Many camping equipment stores sell portable folding stools that you can take along on walks for rest stops. Some models come with a shoulder strap, and others have their own tote bag. You might also find a fold up "cane" seat at pharmacies or in specialty catalogs that can be carried or used much as a cane yet provides a handy seat when you need to rest.

322. **Take individually wrapped moist towelettes (the anti-bacterial kind) when you go out.** They are good for easy clean-up when washroom sinks are inaccessible. Use them when you go out in public and have contact with shopping cart handles, door handles, and public phones—notorious havens for contagious germs. Another option is to use an antibacterial hand sanitizer; these germ-killing gels are great when soap and water are not available.

323. **If you are unable to shake hands using your right hand because of tremors, or another condition, offer your left hand.** If you are unable to offer either hand, simply say, "You'll have to excuse me, I am unable to shake your hand. I offer a smile instead."

Cars and Driving

324. **Find out if you qualify for a disabled parking permit or a disabled license plate,** available to people with health problems or an impaired ability to walk. With the permit, you can park your vehicle in specially designated parking

spaces. In some areas, you also may park at metered stalls without payment and for longer than the posted time limit. Contact your state's Department of Motor Vehicles about obtaining disabled parking privileges. You'll need a signed statement from your physician verifying your need for a temporary or permanent permit and, in some cases, you must periodically recertify your disability.

325. **If you are concerned about your loved one driving safely,** and it is difficult for you to take the car keys away or deny the person the right to drive, talk with your loved one's doctor. Often, a trusted doctor can convince their patient to quit driving when a loved one cannot.

Some doctors may be reluctant to restrict driving privileges. In that case, the Department of Motor Vehicles (DMV) may be your ally. If the person with PD applies for a handicapped parking permit or for disabled plates, she will be required to take a driver's test; the DMV may then revoke the person's driving privileges.**

326. **A No-Start Battery Switch provides peace of mind.** Convincing a loved one that he is unsafe to drive is often a challenging task. By attaching this device to the car battery, you can, with the turn of a knob, disable the car and make it impossible to start. When you want to start the car, simply turn the knob in the opposite direction to enable the battery again. Designed to affect starting only, it will not affect the clock, the radio, or the car's computer settings.*,**

327. **Vehicles with leather or vinyl seats are easier to get into and out of than those with cloth fabric seats.** One way to make sliding in and out of the seat easier is to place a large sheet of plastic, such as a garbage bag or a vinyl drop cloth, on the seat before sitting down.

Travel

Traveling by Car
328. **Take along your personal disabled windshield placard when you travel.** Disabled parking permits are

honored in most states; often, you can use your placard on a rental car or in a car in which you are a passenger. However, some states do not honor disabled placards issued from another state. If you are traveling by car, contact the police department in your destination city to find out about the local ordinances. If you forget to bring your permit with you, you may be able to visit the nearest Department of Motor Vehicles office and request a temporary permit. Don't be surprised if they want to see a doctor's letter certifying your disability or medical condition.

329. **Keep an extra outfit in the car** in case you spill something on your clothing and need to change.

330. **Use a U-shaped inflatable neck pillow to prevent getting a stiff neck from sleeping while sitting up during long car trips.**

331. **If you need to travel with food or medication that needs to be refrigerated,** take along a travel cooler that plugs into your vehicle's cigarette lighter. About the size of a mini-refriger-

ator, it will keep medication, food, and drinks cool while you are driving and maintain that cool without ice for several hours unplugged; AC adaptors are available for home and hotel use. Look for coolers in outdoor and discount stores where camping supplies are sold.*

332. **If you tend to get cold in the car while everyone else is comfortable,** a Car Cozy Car Blanket plugs into your vehicle's cigarette lighter and provides extra warmth. This high-quality fleece blanket is large enough (42 by 58 inches) for two people.*

Making Your Vehicle More Accessible
Many products will make your automobile more accessible and thus make traveling easier, whether across the country or just across town. Here are a few you might find particularly helpful:

333. **Add a portable handle to assist you in getting in or out of vehicle.** If you need help getting in or out of your car, the CarCaddie, a portable handle, straps around the top of your vehicle's window frame to provide a cushion grip. Because it is adjustable and not permanently in-

stalled, it can be moved to other vehicles (although it's not suitable for convertibles or other vehicles without an enclosed window frame).*

334. **The Handybar is a super-strong personal support handle that helps you get in or out of the car with ease.** The removable bar inserts into a U-shaped plate that is installed on your vehicle's door frame. Constructed of a forged steel shaft with a soft, nonslip grip handle, it can be used on either the driver or passenger side and will safely support up to 350 pounds.*

335. **Helping a weak or frail person get into a car with upholstered seats can be difficult. Try tucking a vinyl tablecloth or a plastic garbage bag into the seat.** That way, you'll create a surface that's slippery enough to slide on. Or, purchase one of the many transfer disks available through home health stores. The Flexi-Disc by Phil-E-Slide is made of tough, durable fabric designed to allow the user a better sense of feel and, thus, stability and security when transferring. Simply place the disc on the floor, bed, or car-seat

and use the swivel action to turn into place. The fabric conforms to the user and folds for easy storage between uses.*,**

336. **Seatbelt extender improves ability to grasp, pull, and buckle up.** A seatbelt extender is a piece of seatbelt material, about 8 inches long, with a buckle on the end that clicks into the existing seat belt. Originally designed to provide extra room for larger (over 215 pounds) drivers and passengers, it makes the seatbelt easier to grasp, pull, and buckle for people with arm, shoulder, or strength limitations. Unfortunately, seatbelt extenders are not a universal fit, and some car models do not even offer the device. Some dealers will include the extender when you purchase a new car. Contact your car dealership to see if a seatbelt extender is available for the car you drive.

337. **Ease the transport of a wheelchair or scooter with a variety of lifts and accessibility options for your vehicle.** If you are limited in your ability to get out and about because your wheelchair or scooter is too difficult to transport,

consider adding a lift that picks up the chair and puts it into the vehicle with minimal physical effort. Automatic seats and wheelchair lifts can greatly add to the independence of someone with limited mobility.*

338. **When considering the purchase of a new vehicle,** ask about options and programs available offering discounts and/or rebates for the purchase of adaptive equipment for people with disabilities. Some automobile manufacturers, like Ford and Toyota, have made accessibility options a part of their corporate mission.

Traveling by Air

339. **When making airline reservations, let the ticketing agent know if you have any special needs.** Will you need assistance boarding the plane? Do you require a special meal (low-fat, vegetarian, kosher, etc.)? Do you need an electric cart to get to a connecting flight? Do you need to fly with your oxygen tank? Do you require special seating? (For example, an aisle seat near the restroom if you need to make frequent trips.) If you need more legroom

or have difficulty maneuvering into seats, ask to be assigned to a bulkhead seat, which are at the front of the cabin; these seats are typically reserved for travelers with special needs. Also, keep in mind that, while on board, flight stewards will ask you to stow your cane or walker; let them know in advance if you will need assistance getting up and around in the cabin.

340. **Remember that with heightened airport security, you must present a photo ID** (usually a driver's license) when checking in, so that airport personnel can match your picture ID with the name on the ticket. If you do not have a valid driver's license because of a disability, obtain a picture ID from your state's Department of Motor Vehicles. A small service fee may be charged to obtain a picture ID.

341. **Save energy by making use of the conveniences many airports have for travelers.** When you enter the airport, let a porter call for a wheelchair and carry your bags. Ask, in advance, if he can assist you with your bags to the ticket counter and then take you to the

gate. If you start out with a porter, whom you pay, to take you every step of the way, you will be less stressed and have more energy for the rest of your trip. Once you reach the gate, tell the gate agent if you will need any assistance boarding or during the flight. When you reach your destination, ask the gate agent to call for a porter, and ask the porter to take you from the gate to the baggage carousel, and finally to the taxi stand. It may cost a few dollars for a porter, but it is well worth it.

342. **If you must travel with medication that needs to be refrigerated,** bring along a thermal lunch bag that will hold a few doses of the medication. Insert a cool pack into the bag until you can give it to a flight attendant to refrigerate. It is also a good idea to have a letter from your physician stating that you are taking medication and need to travel with syringes and needles.

Packing

343. **Select the right bag.** Before you plan your next trip, upgrade your luggage. Lightweight, durable Walking Bag lug-

gage helps reduce stress on knees, back, elbows, and shoulders. It rolls in all directions and is very easy to maneuver in crowded places. Available in assorted styles, sizes, and colors, the luggage is made of rugged Teflon-coated 1,200-denier polyester fabric, is very stable, and can be leaned on or sat on. Overall, it takes about one-sixth of the effort to use Walking Bag luggage compared with other types of luggage.*

344. **Soft, cushioned handles and shoulder straps made of neoprene gel, make carrying luggage, briefcase, musical instruments, carts, and the like easier on the hand.** Bright colors serve as a luggage identifier as well.*

345. **Use Ziploc bags (or similar zipper-slide plastic bags) to pack similar items** of clothing together (undergarments in one bag; t-shirts in another) and zip halfway. Then, sit on the bag or squeeze it so that all the air comes out, then zip it tight. You'll find that you can pack your clothing into a smaller, more manageable suitcase. Be sure to pack a change of clothing in

your carry-on bag, just in case your luggage is delayed.

346. **Taking along these items when you travel can really save the day:**

- A collapsible cup and drinking straws

- Cellophane tape

- Paper clips

- Ziploc plastic bags

- A small, folding suitcase

- A tape measure

- An extra wristwatch and pair of eyeglasses

- A calculator

- A small spiral notebook and pencil

- A small flashlight

- Packets of instant coffee, creamer, sweetener, bouillon cubes, and instant soup

- An electric water heater that heats up a cup of coffee or water

347. **Pack your prescriptions and other medications in your carry-on bag.** If you pack them in your suitcase, and the airline misplaces your luggage, you may be stranded without your medicine for at least 24 hours. Also, in case of an emergency, carry an index card with a list of important medical information including your diagnosis, medications, and family and doctors' contact information.

Staying at a Motel or Hotel

348. **Before you go on vacation, contact the hotel where you will be staying and speak with the concierge.** She can make dinner reservations, arrange for play tickets, and provide information about other sights to see that otherwise might be unavailable to you. The concierge service is free, but tips are appreciated.

349. **If you travel with a wheelchair, bring along a length of string that spans the width of your wheelchair or a tape measure.** Before checking

in at a hotel or motel, ask the desk clerk to take the string or measuring tape and use it to measure the width of the door to your room, the bathroom, and the hotel elevator (if applicable). If there is enough clearance, you can check into the hotel with confidence.

350. **When you check into a hotel or motel,** make up a card to leave at the front desk that contains the following information: your name, your room number, the dates of your stay, and a brief description of special assistance you might need in case of emergency. Such an "ability-alert" card will stand out and let hotel and emergency staff know that you need help.

Organizations and Services That Will Make Traveling Easier

351. **The International Association for Medical Assistance to Travelers (IAMAT) is a nonprofit organization that provides important information to travelers with medical concerns.** Travelers can obtain a directory of English-speaking doctors in foreign countries. Updated each year, the directory

lists doctors who have had training in the United States, Great Britain, or Canada. IAMAT also has world immunization charts, malaria risk charts, and world climate charts, and can tell you about the food and water in the countries you plan to visit.*

352. **The International Association of Convention & Visitor Bureaus (IACVB) has an online web directory for travel destinations all over the world.** If you prefer, they also publish a free directory listing the telephone numbers and fax numbers for convention and visitor bureaus for large cities all over the world. Try calling the travel and tourist information bureau of the state you're planning to visit for information on accessibility. Better yet, call the tourism office of the county or city of your destination to find accessible attractions and lodgings. Be persistent.*

353. **The Society for Accessible Travel and Hospitality (SATH) is a nonprofit organization that acts as a clearinghouse for accessible tourism information.** They are in contact with organizations in many countries to promote the

development of facilities for people with disabilities. They publish a quarterly magazine, *Access to Travel.**

354. **Travelin' Talk Network links members with special needs.** If you're still apprehensive about leaving familiar surroundings, become a member of the Travelin' Talk Network. It's a valuable resource for travelers with special needs. Members of the network share knowledge of their hometowns and/or extend a multitude of services to travelers who need help. Whether your wheelchair breaks down or you're trying to locate an accessible vegetarian restaurant, Travelin' Talk members are "your friends away from home."*

355. **Wheelchair Getaways offers wheelchair-accessible van rentals by the day, week, or month.** If an accessible van would make your travel easier, rent one to travel in or at your destination. Vans may be picked up and returned at the Wheelchair Getaways garage location or delivered to your door for a nominal fee.*

RESOURCES

Automotive Accessibility Tools

Bruno Independent Living Aids, Inc.
1780 Executive Drive
P.O. Box 84
Oconomowoc, WI53066
800-882-8183
262-567-4990
www.bruno.com

CarCaddie

Dynamic Living
428 Hayden Station Road
Windsor, CT06095-1302
888-940-0605
www.dynamic-living.com

Car Cozy Blanket

Comfort House
800-359-7701
www.comforthouse.com

Flexi-Disc Flexible Transfer Disk

Phil-E-Slide, Inc.
389 Main Street

Salem, NH03079
866-675-4338
www.phil-e-slide-us.com

Handle Cushion or Gel Handle Grips

TD Innovations
18217 Crystal Street
Grass Valley, CA95949
530-477-9780
www.shorelinecases.com

Handybar

Dynamic Living
428 Hayden Station Road
Windsor, CT06095-1302
888-940-0605
www.dynamic-living.com

Lightweight, Wheeled Luggage

SWANY America Corp.
EZ-Swany Division
115 Corporate Drive
Johnstown, NY, 12095
800-237-9269
518-725-2026
www.ezswany.com

No-Start Battery Switch

Ageless Design, Inc.
12633159th Court North
Jupiter, FL33478-6669
800-752-3238
www.alzstore.com

Organizations and Services That Will Make Traveling Easier

The International Association of Convention &
 Visitor Bureaus (IACVB)
2025 M Street NW,
Suite 500 Washington, DC20036
202-296-7888
www.iacvb.org

International Association for Medical Assistance
 to Travelers (IAMAT)
IAMAT USA
1623 Military Road #279
Niagara Falls, NY14304-1745
716-754 4883
www.iamat.org

Society for Accessible Travel & Hospitality
 (SATH)
New York, NY10016
212-447-7284

www.sath.org

Travelin' Talk Network
Access-Able Travel Source
www.travelintalk.net

Wheelchair Getaways
P.O. Box 605
Versailles, KY40383
800-536-5518
859-873-8039
www.wheelchairgetaways.com

Thermoelectric Coolers

Coleman Corporation
800-835-3278
www.coleman.com

About the Author

Shelley Peterman Schwarz and her husband Dave live in Madison, Wisconsin. They've been married since 1969 and are enjoying being the parents of two adult children, Jamie and Andrew, and grandparents to Jamie's little girl, Jordan. Jamie and her husband David live and work in Chicago. Andrew and his wife, Ronit, live in Tucson where Andrew is in graduate school at the University of Arizona.

At the time of her multiple sclerosis (MS) diagnosis in 1979, Shelley was working part-time as a teacher of the deaf. Two years later, due to the effects of progressive MS, she retired. In 1985, when a story she wrote appeared in *Inside MS,* the magazine of the National Multiple Sclerosis Society, a new career was born. Since then Shelley has published more than 450 articles. She also has received numerous awards, including the Mother of the Year from the Wisconsin Chapter of the National MS Society and the Spirit of the American Woman Award from JC Penney, and she was named a Woman of Distinction by the YWCA.

Shelley's nationally syndicated column, "Making Life Easier," appears in numerous newspapers and magazines internationally, including

SpecialLiving, Inside MS, Real Living with MS, Arthritis Today, and *Humana Active Outlook.* Her tips are available on numerous web sites as well. In 1997, the National Arthritis Foundation, Inc., commissioned Shelley to write *250 Tips for Making Life with Arthritis Easier* based on her "Making Life Easier" column. More *Making Life Easier* books followed. (See a list of additional books by Shelley on page ix.)

In 1995, Shelley self-published a book entitled, *Blooming Where You're Planted: Stories from the Heart.* The previously published essays chronicle her journey of change and self-discovery following her MS diagnosis. A professional speaker, Shelley's philosophy of life is to find solutions to whatever problems she faces and to help others do the same. Her motivational and inspirational keynotes and workshops help audiences see challenges in their lives as opportunities for personal growth. She shares her message of hope and teaches audiences how to "bloom wherever they're planted."

Visit www.MeetingLifesChallenges.com to contact Shelley, subscribe to her free e-zine, to read her blog and personal essays, or to learn about her teleclasses.

A

'Ability-alert' card, *204*

AbilityOne Company, *47-48, 115-116, 147, 184*

ABLEDATA, *14*

Access to Recreation, Inc., *150*

Access with Ease, Inc., *47, 49, 67, 151*

Active Forever, *51, 69, 116*

Adaptation, importance of, *2*

Adaptations by Adrian, *66*

Adapting the Home for the Physically Challenged, *45*

Adaptive devices or equipment, *9, 18, 27, 102-103, 115*

   See also Assistive devices,

Advantage Rail, *31*

Advocacy, *7*

Ageless Design, Inc., *45, 48, 91, 93, 147, 208*

AgeNet, Inc., *117*

Air travel,

   airport conveniences, *199*

   luggage, *200, 208*

   medications, *200*

   packing tips, *200, 202*

   photo ID, *199*

   special needs notification, *199*

Allegro Medical, *147, 184*

Allergies, *179*

Allergy medications, *155*

Always Something Brilliant, *151*

American Health Care Apparel, Ltd., *66*

American Parkinson's Disease Association (APDA), Inc., *13, 155, 183*

Amigo Mobility International, Inc., *149*

Amplivox Sound Systems, *93*

Ankle-foot orthotic (APO) brace, *66, 122*

Antidepressant medications, *5*
Appetite, loss of, *4*
Assistance Dogs United Campaign, *146*
Assistive devices,
    benefits of, *9, 42, 121, 127, 131, 133*
    sources for, *182-183*
Attainment Company, Inc., *49, 91*
Audio books, *137-138*
Automatic Faucet, *45*
Automatic Telephone 'Hanger Upper', *83, 85*

B
Baby food, *111*
Backrest, *177*
Bathroom, safety guidelines,
    faucets, *35-36*
    grab bars, *31-32*
    information resources, *45, 47*
    overview of, *35-36*
    shower doors, *29*
    water heater thermostat, *22*
Bed Handles, *47*

Bedroom, safety guidelines,
    bed sheets, *42*
    information resources, *47-48*
    pillow support, *177*
    repositioning guidelines, *40, 42*
    set up of, *39-40*
    turning over in bed, *42-43*
Bed Specs, *138, 147*
Bob Hope Parkinson Research Center, *14*
Book clubs, *135*
Books, as information resource, *15, 17, 117*
Bruce Medical Supply, *47, 116*
Bruno Independent Living Aids, Inc., *18, 51, 206*
Buck & Buck, *67*

C
Canes, *9, 121, 127, 130-131*
Canine Companions for Independence, *146*
Carbon monoxide detectors, *22, 24*
CarCaddie, *195, 207*

Card games, tips for, *142, 144, 149, 151*

Caregivers,
   basic concepts for, *11, 13*
   patient repositioning guidelines, *40, 42*
   support groups for, *17*
   verbal cues, *13*

Cars,
   accessibility tools, *195, 197, 199, 206-207*
   adaptive equipment, *9, 197*
   disabled license plate, *191*
   No-Start Battery Switch, *191, 193, 208*
   parking permits, *191, 193*
   seatbelts, *197*
   seating material, *193, 195, 197*

Change-A-Robe, *60, 67*

Chattervox, *93*

Chewing, *5, 107*

Choking, *109, 111*

Chronic conditions, information resources, *17*

Church, as medical supply resource, *183*

Chux, *175*

Clothing,
   adaptive, *62, 64, 66-67*
   selection factors, *59-60*

Cognitive deficits, *122*

Cold medicines, *155*

Comfort House, *207*

Commodes, *36, 52*

Communicating,
   information resources, *91, 93*
   lines of communication, *87, 89, 91*
   problems with, *73-74, 122*
   speaking tips, *74, 76, 78-79*
   technological aids, *82-83, 85*
   writing tips, *85, 87*

Complete Directory for People with Disabilities, 2005 Edition, The, *15*

Compresses, *175*

ConAgra Foods, *117*

Concentration difficulties, *122*
   improvement exercises, *144, 146*

Confusion, *43, 62*

Constipation, *179*

Consumer's Guide to Home Adaptation, *43*

Cooking utensils, *100*

Coolers, *193, 195, 210*

Coping strategies, *2, 4*

Cordless telephones, *29*

Coughing, *107, 109*

Cozy Car Blanket, *195, 207*

Creative Designs, *67*

Credit card safety, *188-189*

Cutting boards, *32, 51*

D

Daily activities participation in, *11*
   supportive help with, *9*

Dancing, *127*

D.C. Distributors, Inc., *116*

DDS Products, LLC, *67*

Delusions, *11, 162*

Dementia, *43*

Deming Designs Inc., *150*

Demos Medical Publishing, *15*

Dental care, *55, 57*

Department of Motor Vehicles (DMV), *191, 193*

Depression, *4-5*

Dereiko-Teutsch & Associates, *119*

Diagnosis, *2, 4-5*

Dietary supplements, *155*

Dining out, *2, 189*

Disabilities Resources Monthly, *15*

Doctor-patient relationship, *4-5, 39, 154-155*
   See also Physicians,

Documentation, *159*
   See also Recordkeeping,

Doorbell, *27, 29*

Door stop sign, *25, 27, 48*

Doubleday Large Print, *149*

Dressing,
   aids, *62, 64*
   clothing adaptations, *62, 64*
   clothing selection, *59-60*
   footwear, *64, 66*
   grooming, *54-55, 57, 59*
   hosiery, *64, 66*
   information resources, *66-67, 69-71*
   tips for, *60, 62*

Dressing stick, *64*

Driveway sensors, *24, 48*

Driving safety, *7, 188, 191, 193*

  See also Car safety,

Dry mouth syndrome, *105, 107, 172, 174*

Dycem Limited, *116*

Dynamic Living, *49, 147, 183, 207*

Dysphagia, *103*

E

Easy Street Co., *47, 52, 70, 115, 146, 186*

Eating,

  see Mealtime,

Eazykey Ltd., *48*

Embarrassment, *2*

Emergency or emergencies,

  provisions, *22, 24*

  response systems, *179*

  services, special needs notification, *13*

Emotional energy, *2*

Employment status, *7*

Empowerment,

  information resources, *146-147, 149-151, 153*

  leisure and recreational activities, *135, 137-138, 141-142, 144, 146*

mobility and exercise, *122, 124, 126-127, 130-131, 133, 135*

  significance of, *121-122*

Encouragement, importance of, *11*

Energy,

  conservation, *9*

  level, *5, 7, 95*

Epiphany Design, *67*

Errands, *188-189, 191*

Everyday tasks, *9, 11*

Exercise program, *5, 9, 11, 122, 124, 126-127, 130-131, 133, 135*

F

Facial expression, *5, 73-74*

Family Caregiver Alliance, *17*

Family roles, *4, 11*

  See also Caregivers,

Fear, *5, 7*

Flexibility, importance of, *7*

Floor coverings, *19, 43*

Focus, *5, 11*

Food preparation,

  cooking utensils, *100*

  finger foods, *102*

  jar opening tips, *98, 100, 116*

Prep Taxi, *100, 119*
Food supplements, *105*
Food thickeners, *116-117*
Footwear, *64, 66, 177*
4-in-1 Fleece Blanket, *138, 146*
Frustration, *5, 73, 78, 122*
Furniture,
    arrangement of, *19-20*
    selection factors, *43*

G

Gait, *126-127*
Games, playing tips, *142, 144, 149*
Gel Handle Grips, *207*
Golden Cuisine, *98, 117*
Go Talk, *82*
Grab bars, *29, 31-32, 40*
Grocery services,
on-line, *96, 119*
Grocery shopping, *95-96*
Guardian Safe-T-Pole, *31*
Guilt, dealing with, *2*

H

Hallucinations, *11, 162, 175*
Handi-Robe, *60*
Handle Cushion, *207*

Handshake guidelines, *191*
Handwriting, *74*
Handybar, *195, 207*
Healthcare directives, *159*
Health Craft Products, Inc., *51-52*
Health Watch Inc., *179, 183*
Heating pad, *175*
Herbal remedies, *155*
Home accessibility, *9*
Home health agencies, *183*
Home healthcare, *175, 177, 179, 182-183*
Home safety guidelines,
    emergency response systems, *179*
    information resources, *45, 47-49, 51-52, 89*
    overview of, *19-20, 22, 24-25, 27, 29, 31-32, 35-36, 39-40, 42-43*
Hopelessness, *4*
Hosiery, *54-55, 57, 59, 64, 66, 177*
Hospitalization, *174-175*
Humor, importance of, *2, 4*

I

IAMAT USA, *208*

Improvements Catalog, *186*

Incontinence, nighttime, *39*

Independent living centers (ILCs), *17*

Independent living skills training, *7*

Independent Living Aids, Inc., *69, 147, 149*

Independent Living Center (ILC), *7*

Information resources, *1-2, 5, 7, 13-15, 17-18, 45, 47-49, 51-52, 66-67, 69-71, 91, 93, 115-117, 119-120, 146-147, 149-151, 153, 155, 166, 183-184, 186, 204, 206-208, 210*

Intercom system, *27, 29, 48*

International Association for Medical Assistance to Travelers (IAMAT), *204, 208*

International Association of Convention & Visitor Bureaus (IACVB), *206, 208*

J

Jar opening tips, *98, 100, 116*

Jewelry,
medical ID, *179, 182, 184*
vibrating locket, *170, 186*

Jobst USA, *70*

K

Keyless entry, *27*

Kitchen, safety guidelines, *32, 35*

L

Lamps, touch-sensitive, *20, 22, 52*

Language impairment, information resources, *91*

L-Bow Mittens, *146*

Leg cramps, *177*

Legal issues, *159*

Leisure activities, *135, 137-138, 141-142, 144, 146*

Levadopa, *174*

License plate, *191*

Life with Ease, *51*

Lifeline, *179, 184*

Lighting,
hands-free, *131*

safety guidelines, *19-20, 22, 43*

touch-sensitive lamps, *20, 22, 52*

Liquid diet, *105, 113*

Living with Low Vision A Resource Guide for People with Sight Loss, *17*

Luggage, *208*

Luminaud, Inc., *93*

M

Maddak, Inc., *117, 119, 151*

Masked faces, *73*

Massage, *43, 76*

Maxi Aids, Inc., *115*

Meal delivery services, *117, 119*

Meals on Wheels, *98, 119*

Meals on Wheels Association of America, *98*

Mealtime,
 adaptive devices at, *102-103, 115*
 drooling, *109*
 eating utensils, *100, 102, 119*
 food consistency and texture, *109, 111, 113, 116-117*
 food preparation, *116, 119*
 grocery shopping, *96, 119*
 information resources, *115-117, 119-120*
 meal delivery, *98, 117, 119*
 meal planning and preparation, *95-96, 98, 100, 102*
 napkins, *103, 117*
 placemats, *102, 116*
 plates, *117*
 swallowing difficulties, coping strategies, *103, 105, 107, 109*
 swallowing pills and vitamins, *113, 115*

Med-Diet Laboratories, *117*

MedGlider System, *170*

Medical alert systems, *179, 183-184*

Medical care,
 doctors' appointments, *157, 161-162, 165*
 home healthcare, *175, 177, 179, 182-183*
 information resources, *155, 183-184, 186*

medical alert systems, *183-184*

medical ID jewelry, *184*

medical supplies, *184*

medical tests, *165*

medications, *165-166, 168, 170, 172, 174-175, 186*

patient education, *155*

Patient's Bill of Rights, *155*

physician, selection factors, *154-155*

recordkeeping, *155, 157, 159, 161, 165, 183*

research, *159, 161*

MedicAlert, *179, 182*

Medical journals, *155*

Medical supplies, *182, 184*

Medication,

absorption of, *105*

administration of, *4, 172, 174*

antidepressants, *5*

diet and, *174*

dosage, *162, 166, 168, 172*

information resources, *166, 186*

mood changes, *174*

packing for travel, *200, 202*

patient education, *155*

pill splitting, *172*

prescription abbreviations, *166*

prescription log, *157*

recordkeeping guidelines, *159, 166, 168, 170*

schedule for, *168, 170, 174*

side effects, *165, 175*

sleep patterns and, *162*

swallowing guidelines, *105, 113, 115, 170, 172*

travel preparations, *193, 195, 200, 202, 210*

Medic ID International, *184*

Medicine Program, The, *182, 186*

Meditation, *9, 11*

MediUSA, *70*

Meeting Life's Challenges, *17*

Memory impairment,

improvement exercises, *144, 146*

management strategies, *122*

Mental energy, *2*

Michael J. Fox Foundation for

Parkinsons' Research, the, *14*

Mindfulness classes, *11*

Mind-set, significance of, *1-2, 4-5, 7, 9, 11*

Mobility, *7, 9, 130-131, 133*

Modifications,
  information resources, *45, 47-49, 51-52*
  types of, *19-20, 22, 24-25, 27, 29, 31-32, 35-36, 39-40, 42-43*

Motion detector lights, *22*

MotionPAD, *24, 49*

N

Napkins, *117*

Napping, *5*

National Council on Independent Living, *17*

National Federation of the Blind, *135, 137, 153*

National Institute on Disability and Rehabilitation Research, *14*

National Institutes of Health, *183*

National Kitchen & Bath Association, *45*

National Library of Medicine, *159, 183*

National Library Service for the Blind and Physically Handicapped, *14, 151*

National Parkinson's Foundation, Inc. (NPF), *14, 155*

National Rehabilitation Information Center (NARIC), *14*

Natural Access, *150*

Neck support, *177, 193*

Newsletters, as information resource, *15, 17*

Newspapers, Talking, *135, 137, 153*

Nonverbal cues, *73*

North Coast Medical, Inc., *120*

No-Start Battery Switch, *191, 193, 208*

O

Occupational therapist (OT), functions of, *7, 9, 25, 154*

Orthopedic specialist, functions of, *124, 154*

Outdoor accessibility, *133, 135, 150*

Outings, *188-189, 191*

P

Pain relievers, *155*

Parking permits, *191, 193*

Parkinson's Action Network, *15*

Parkinson's Disease Foundation, Inc., *15*

Park Surgical Co., Inc., *93*

Patience, importance of, *7*

Patient Assistance Programs, *182*

Patient,
   advocacy, *7*
   education, *155*

Patient's Bill of Rights, *155*

Paws with a Cause, *146*

Peer support, *7*

Personal care attendants, *7*

Pharmacists, functions of, *154, 166, 168*

Phil-E-Slide, *133, 197, 207*

Phil-E-Slide, USA, *150, 207*

Physiatrists, functions of, *154*

Physical energy, *2*

Physical therapist (PT), functions of, *7, 9, 11, 25, 122, 154, 177*

Physician,
   bedside manner of, *154*
   recommendations, *155*
   referrals, *154*
   relationship with, *4-5, 39, 154-155*
   selection factors, *154-155*

Physician's Desk Reference (PDR), *166, 183*

Planet Media Group, *183*

Plastic chair protectors, *43, 49*

Plates, *117*

Pneumonia, *109*

Positive attitude, importance of, *4-5*

Power of attorney, *159*

Pow-R-Grips handles, *32, 35, 49*

Prioritizing, importance of, *5*

Prism glasses, *138, 147*

Products for Seniors, *52*

Professional organizations, as information resource, *13-14*

    See also specific organizations,

Psychiatrist, functions of, *154*

Psychologist, functions of, *154*

Psychotherapy, benefits of, *5, 174*

R

Ramps, *29*

Range-of-motion exercises, *9*

Reachers, *20, 49*

Reading strategies, *135, 137-138*

Recordkeeping, *155, 157, 159, 161, 165, 183*

Recreation, outdoor, *133, 135*

Red Cross, *183*

Referrals, *7*

Relaxation strategies, *141-142, 147*

Remote controls, *141, 147*

Research, sources for, *159, 161, 166*

Resources for Rehabilitation, *17*

Rest, importance of, *2*

Rugs, safety guidelines, *19*

S

Sadness, *4*

Safe-T-Pole, *52*

Salvation Army, *183*

Sammons Preston Rolyan, *47-48, 69, 115-116, 147, 149, 184*

Scooters, as assistive device, *9, 131, 133, 177, 197*

Seatbelts, *197*

Self-consciousness, *2*

Self-pity, *4*

Senior centers, *183*

Service dogs, *133, 135, 146*

Shopping trips, *96, 119, 189*

Shower, safety guidelines,

    grab bars, *29, 31-32*

    overview, *20*

Silvert's, *71*

Sinemet, *174*

Sleep patterns, *5, 162*

Smarthome, *48*

Smell, loss of, *22, 24*

Smoke detectors, *22, 24*

Society for Accessible Travel & Hospitality (SATH), *204, 206, 208*
Solutions Catalog, *49, 119*
Specialized Care Co., *70*
Speech amplifiers, *82*
Speech problems,
  information resources, *91*
  types of, *4, 13*
Speech-to-speech relay, *93*
Spoons, *119*
Stairlift, *31-32, 51*
Stairs, safety guidelines,
  railings, *29, 31*
  types of, *29, 124, 126*
Storage, safety guidelines, *20, 32, 40*
Stress reduction strategies, *2, 11, 78*
Stretching regimens, *9*
STSnews, *93*
Suits Me Swimwear, *69*
Sunrise Medical (North American Operations), *47, 52*
Super Pole System, *31, 52*
Support groups,
  benefits of, *5, 7, 13, 174*
  as information resource, *159, 161*
Support poles, *31, 51*
Swallowing difficulties,
  diagnosis, *103, 105*
  impact of, *5, 74*
  information resources, *115, 119*
  mealtime guidelines, *103, 105*
  medications, *113*
  reduction strategies, *105, 107, 109*
SWANY America Corp., *208*
Swimming program, *9*
Swimsuits, *60, 69*

T
Tai Chi, *9*
Talking Book Program, *137-138, 151*
Talking Pill Bottle, *166, 186*
TD Innovations, *207*
Telecommunications Relay Service, *87, 89*
Telephones, *82-83, 91, 93*
Television-watching strategies, *138, 141-142, 147*
Thermo pellets, *120*

Thermometer, digital, *175*

Thomas Fetterman, Inc., *151*

Time management, *5*

Total Living Company, *49*

Transport chairs, *9*

Travel,

by air, *199-200*

assistive agencies, *204, 206*

by car, *193, 195, 197, 199*

information resources, *204, 206-208, 210*

packing, *200, 202*

Travelin' Talk Network, *206, 210*

TravelSox, *70*

Tremors, *2, 31, 57, 70, 102, 126*

U

Uncle's Games, *149*

U.S. Department of Education, as information resource, *14*

United Way, *98*

U-shaped handles, *29, 31*

V

Verbal cues, *13, 79*

Visiting Nurse Service, *183*

Visual impairment, information resources, *17, 151, 153*

reading strategies, *135, 137-138, 149*

stair safety, *31*

television-watching strategies, *138, 141-142, 147*

Vitamins, *113, 115, 155*

Voice projection, *5*

W

Walkers, *9, 121, 131, 133*

Walking exercise program, *9, 122, 124, 126*

Walking stick, *131*

Wandering, *162*

Weather conditions, walking guidelines, *130-131*

Wheelchair, *177, 197, 202, 204*

Wheelchair,

Wheelchair,

Wheelchair Getaways, *206, 210*

Wheelchairs,

clearance for, *25*

lifts, *197*

ramps, *29*

safety guidelines, *2, 4,
9, 121, 131, 177, 202, 204*

Y
Yoga, *9*

Z
Zackaroos, *69*
Zapper Adapter, *22*
Zipper ties, *60, 71*

Books For ALL Kinds of Readers

At ReadHowYouWant we understand that one size does not fit all types of readers. Our innovative, patent pending technology allows us to design new formats to make reading easier and more enjoyable for you. This helps improve your speed of reading and your comprehension. Our EasyRead printed books have been optimized to improve word recognition, ease eye tracking by adjusting word and line spacing as well as minimizing hyphenation. Our EasyRead SuperLarge editions have been developed to make reading easier and more accessible for vision-impaired readers. We offer Braille and DAISY formats of our books and all popular E-Book formats.

We are continually introducing new formats based upon research and reader preferences. Visit our web-site to see all of our formats and learn how you can Personalize our books for yourself or as gifts. Sign up to Become A (RHYW) Registered Reader.

www.readhowyouwant.com

LaVergne, TN USA
01 March 2010
174584LV00003B/50/P